Integrating Modern Medicine and Traditional Chinese Medicine

Lecture Series by Tsun-Nin Lee, M.D.

Volume One: Acupuncture

About the Author

Dr. Tsun-Nin Lee received his B.A. from Columbia College and M.D. from New York University School of Medicine. He received his postgraduate training in medicine at the University Hospital of Jacksonville in Florida. In 1975, he became a diplomate of Advanced Chinese Acupuncture at the Hong Kong Acupuncture Institute. That same year, he was awarded the Certificate of Competence from the Chinese Medical Institute in Hong Kong. He is the permanent honorary director of the Cultural Center of Chinese Medicine in Hong Kong. He is a member of the Chinese Association of the Integration of Traditional and Western Medicine. Dr. Lee has practiced and taught integrative medicine for more than 35 years. He is the director of the Academy of Pain Research, which first organized a prototype acupuncture course in 1979, the forerunner of the Comprehensive Training Course on Acupuncture for Physicians. In 2003, Dr. Lee designed and established the Comprehensive Training Course on Herbal Medicine for Physicians to complement the acupuncture training program. Thousands of physicians have benefited from Dr. Lee's courses in integrating modern and traditional Chinese medicine.

Dr. Tsun-Nin Lee is the proponent of the thalamic neuron theory, which was published in a series of papers between 1976 and 2002 in *Medical Hypothesis*, to explain the phenomena and principles of traditional Chinese medicine from the modern scientific point of view, as well as to shed light on many enigmas encountered in the practice of modern medicine.

Introduction

The contents of this book feature the transcripts of an audio lecture series presented at the beginning of the Comprehensive Training Course on Acupuncture for Physicians to familiarize the participants with the concepts of traditional Chinese medicine (TCM).

The major stumbling block for modern physicians in appreciating the true value of TCM largely stems from their failure to comprehend the seemingly abstruse terminology of TCM. Many of the difficult-to-grasp principles of TCM relate primarily to the functions of the central nervous system, the complexities of which have so far eluded the full understanding of modern scientists. With the help of the thalamic neuron theory, a hypothesis propounded by the author in three separate installments spanning the last several decades, a reasonable explanation is now at hand to reconcile the apparent differences between modern medicine and TCM.
This book delves into only some of the many theoretical and practical aspects of acupuncture, an important component of TCM. This book represents the initial effort in the daunting task of integrating Eastern and Western systems of healing.
Converting the audio lectures into print will, perhaps, allow a greater distribution of the information in this course to a greater number of health professionals, thus helping to promote a deeper understanding of this highly valuable tool for healing in a variety of clinical disorders.

Table of Contents

Chapter One – Introduction and Philosophical Approach to the Learning of Acupuncture

Welcome to the *Comprehensive Training Course on Acupuncture for Physicians*. If you think of me as Mr. Roarke on the old TV show "Fantasy Island" and that as soon as you step on the island, you will have all of your wildest dreams fulfilled, that you will be the very best doctor there is, curing all sorts of incurable diseases and getting rid of chronic, intractable, painful conditions with just a few acupuncture treatments after you have spent maybe five or six months studying acupuncture, then you may be in for a disappointment. If, on the other hand, you want to learn about traditional Chinese medicine and acupuncture, and apply that knowledge to treat your patients and help them to alleviate their pain and suffering in a more efficient way, and to successfully treat a number of clinical conditions that have been well known to be intractable to modern medical therapy, then the goal is eminently attainable.

Acupuncture is a technique that requires both skill and knowledge, and you'll need to practice in order to achieve a certain level of competence. It is for this reason that we have designed the course the way it is, so that when you come to San Francisco for the face-to-face didactic and hands-on sessions, you will have plenty of opportunity to do hands-on practice throughout the entire period. There will be different kinds of hands-on experiences from day to day, including point location, body acupuncture techniques, auricular acupuncture techniques, some of the non-invasive needleless techniques such as moxibustion, ultrasound, electrical stimulation, cupping, etc.

Also included will be diagnostic techniques used in traditional Chinese medicine and acupuncture such as ear diagnosis, tongue diagnosis, pulse diagnosis, diagnosis by history, physical examination based on the traditional theories and so on. This period will constitute Stage 2 of Phase 1. We are now in Stage 1, the purpose of which is to prepare you well for Stage 2. That's why we ask you to listen to a number of CDs, followed by viewing of DVDs. The CDs are designed to provide you with the foundations of traditional Chinese medicine and acupuncture, so that you can make good sense out of the rest of the program. The CDs may refer to some of the text that has been provided to you, in order for you to follow easily. The video portion contains the instructional DVD, which teaches you how to find commonly used acupuncture points. As you watch that DVD or after you have done so, you should make an attempt to find points on people around you such as your parents, your spouse, your children, your friends, your in-laws (well, maybe that's not such a good idea), plus any other strangers that might come your way who permit you to do that to them.

Anyway, this should be a very good experience for you because if you make a mistake, you can afford to do so. When you come to the didactic session during Stage 2, you'll have plenty of opportunities to be corrected in point location, making sure everything you do is up to par. Without a doubt, during this phase of learning, you might wonder whether you are finding the points correctly. Questions that you encounter during this experience will be answered subsequently, during the hands-on, face-to-face session. Additionally, we also have a DVD showing the way acupuncture is done.

But at this stage, please try not to move ahead and insert needles before the training, because you will have that opportunity when you come to San Francisco.

Before you listen to each disc, we suggest you first take the pre-test, to determine how much knowledge you already have about acupuncture. This is also a good gauge to determine how much knowledge you don't have. Later, after the listening to the audio, you can retest your knowledge with the post-test to determine how much you have learned.

Each hour of lecture is followed by a test, the post-test. You can send us the test results for both the pre-tests and post-tests, along with any questions you may have regarding the contents of those lectures.

Subsequently, we will make the test scores available, for you to gauge your progress. On top of that, we will collect your questions to answer during the face-to-face sessions, screening them ahead of time to make sure the questions relate to the general content of the course in order to save time, because no doubt everybody has individual questions. If we are able to answer the questions in a collective manner, then most of the questions will be answered to the satisfaction of all our participants. Needless to say, you will still have the opportunity to ask questions individually when we have the face-to-face meeting. Armed with the knowledge you gain from Stage 2, you will be given multiple DVD instructions to take home with you, so you can study at home. These DVDs should be returned when you come back for Phase 2, and if you do not plan to come back for Phase 2 this time, please return the DVDs to us when the study period is finished, within the time frame specified. Phase 2 will emphasize clinical problem-solving, when you will have the opportunity to study different specific disorders relating to different fields in medicine.

The instructors or faculty members will then demonstrate their approaches, and you will have the opportunity to actually put the knowledge to use amongst yourselves, such as using the diagnostic techniques – pulse diagnosis, tongue diagnosis, taking the history from one another and then actually apply the knowledge in an actual clinical setting. The faculty will also conduct what is known as a clinical run, as if you are coming to their clinics to observe them treat a patient using whatever approach that is appropriate for that particular clinical situation. Hands-on experience will also continue throughout Phase 2, under supervision of course. And this will facilitate the learning of acupuncture both in terms of the modality and the clinical application. In between the end of the didactic session of Stage 2 and Phase 2, of course the home study DVDs will show you some additional techniques, such as intramuscular stimulation, non-invasive acupuncture modalities, as well as the very useful injection techniques. For the few of you who elect not to take Phase 2 together with Phase 1 or unable to take Phase 2 because of scheduling problems, we strongly recommend you to take Phase 2 the first opportunity you have, so that what you have learned will be consolidated in your mind. That is probably the most efficient way of acquiring the knowledge and skill necessary to be a successful practitioner of acupuncture.

Now let us turn our attention to the philosophy of learning and performing acupuncture.

The first question we might want to ask is "Why do we need to learn acupuncture and why now?"

Some of you may say, it is high time to learn acupuncture because patients demand to have this kind of service at a physician's office.

Others of you might say, well, it is because now it is economically feasible to incorporate this technique into one's practice, as all the major insurance companies are actually paying for acupuncture service, including some of the HMOs, which recognize this is a better way to provide better health care to patients at large. In addition to the health insurance companies' reimbursing for this service, many patients are actually willing to pay out-of-pocket for this particular treatment. They have been doing so for many many years. Even in the Workers Compensation system such as the one in California, one will be able to get reimbursed for acupuncture, although generally speaking, the reimbursement rate for the Workers Compensation system is lower than the private health care system. Therefore, incorporating acupuncture into one's practice makes good economic sense.

Others of you could offer that by virtue of the nature of this particular modality of treatment, you will be able to spend more time with patients, which you are not able to do under ordinary circumstances, being overwhelmed with patient care under the umbrella of the HMOs. And you miss that interaction with your patients. The rendering of acupuncture treatment will allow you to do so because as you are providing the treatment while doing the needling, you will be able to talk to your patient, and communicating with them about their problems facilitates bonding with your patients. It is not unlike the patient going to a bartender or a hairdresser and then spilling their guts about their personal problems except, of course, as professionals we should do much better than the bartender or the hairdresser.

Others of you would respond by saying that you are looking for alternatives to the conventional way that medical care is delivered. You will find this approach more satisfying for helping patients who are using drug therapy, for example, for chronic pain. You will be able to alleviate sleep problems without prescribing sleeping pills, and you will be able to lift them out of their depression without having to prescribe heavy duty SSRIs, etc.

All of these are valid reasons. Note that I said valid reasons, not the best reasons. In fact one of the best reasons for you to learn acupuncture is to improve your knowledge of Western modern medicine by arming yourself with what you learn in acupuncture and traditional Chinese medicine.

You will, in fact, be able to understand and use Western modern medicine better. You will be able to gain more rational understanding of some of the things that we are doing in modern medicine. You will be able to predict certain side-effects in association with drug therapy. You will be able to avoid certain pitfalls of some of the therapeutic regimens we use in our practices.

In other words, if you were to completely stop practicing traditional Chinese medicine, herbal medicine or acupuncture, you would still be able to apply this knowledge in a very constructive manner to modern medical treatments. You will understand what I mean as we proceed further into the course.

Almost all of the major medical centers and university medical schools nowadays offer some sort of alternative medical education, or they have established an alternative medicine department or center. This trend began more or less around the mid-1990s, after the publication of the work of David Eisenberg, et al. of Harvard School of Medicine, where they presented data indicating that close to one fourth of the US adult population obtained alternative medical treatments from practitioners outside of the mainstream of medicine. And in fact they were willing to pay all related expenses out of their own pockets. At the time, this came as a major surprise to many American physicians. Suddenly, everyone realized that there was a major economic wave underway that, if they didn't catch it, they would be bowled over, so to speak, by it.

And from then on, many universities got themselves involved in the provision of alternative therapies, offering at least some fragmentary approach to the study of alternative or complementary medicine in the medical education curriculum. This is essentially a consumer-driven phenomenon, because no one wakes up one day and says, "Well, what kind of treatments are we offering our patients? I don't think we are offering the best medicine." In the mainstream, doctors are very complacent about what they do, and not until they find out that patients are going to all these alternative practitioners without their knowledge and are in fact willing to foot the bill themselves did they act on this wave of patients' sentiment. Getting them to think, 'Well, perhaps there is something not quite right with the way we deliver medical care', and hence this complete turnaround of attitude towards non-conventional therapies. Basically due to this unstoppable revolution, everybody is now trying to jump on the bandwagon of alternative, complementary, integrative medicine.

But more than a quarter of century ago, I was in fact the driver of this bandwagon, except it wasn't a bandwagon then; it was just an old Model T at best, without all the bells and whistles. I was in fact offering rides to my colleagues, telling them, "Look, if you have a patient with this problem or your relatives have certain intractable painful conditions, I'd be willing to provide treatments for them for free, in fact, so that you know how good this treatment modality may be."

When I was doing that, I thought I was offering to them rides on this bandwagon, but what they perceived was that I was just taking them for a ride. They didn't take me up on it, and I had essentially no referrals whatsoever from physicians. All my patients were referred to me by other patients I had treated; basically my practice was sustained by word of mouth. As you recall, in those days you couldn't even advertise, you couldn't even put up an ad in a newspaper or phone book to indicate what specialty you were in. In fact, at one point I was invited by a claim-men's group, the group of adjusters working for insurance companies' workers compensation system to a meeting, to give a talk. Later on, some adjusters came to see me, and I told them that I was in fact willing to treat their patients and if I did not have results, they shouldn't pay me. And you know how many patients I got as a result? Zero.

4

So when I first started my medical practice focusing on pain management and acupuncture, I made a very sincere effort to convince my colleagues. I even gave professional courtesy to a dentist who practiced in my neighborhood. I recall this gentleman had three major problems: Hypertension, both systolic and diastolic; a symptom complex consistent with gastroesophageal reflux disease or GERD; and last but not least, erectile dysfunction. This gentleman had a divorce a couple of years before he consulted me, had a new girlfriend at the time, and he had this particular problem that he really wanted to take care of. Remember, in those days, Viagra was not available. He also had a rather typical Type A personality, so I did something rather unconventional besides putting in the needles in a traditional way using the appropriate acupuncture points: I used a specific point at the tip of his nose, and that point represents the external genitalia, believe it or not. And of course that teaches you never to rub noses with strangers. In any event, I tried to be innovative: Since he had a HOT personality, something COLD might be appropriate. So, I put an ice cube on the tip of his nose, in conjunction with regular acupuncture, and I euphemized this technique as "ice cube puncture." But it worked. A certain part of his anatomy that was originally as soft as water became as hard as ice and although I wasn't able to change his personality and turn him into a Cool Hand Luke, I was able to manage to turn him into a hot-nosed Jim. In combination with other treatments, I was able to return his blood pressure to normal levels, and get rid of all the GERD symptoms that he had.

And what did I get out from this experience? Monetarily, I got nothing. He did take me to a medium-priced Italian restaurant so I had a good time, and since he did so well, he actually referred his ex-wife and his daughter to me for treatment, also without charge, of course. And I took care of both of their health problems.

Altogether, I probably gave the family over 40 sessions of treatments free of charge. But when I subsequently referred to him a relative of mine for very limited dental work, he gave us a 20% discount, a very generous offer from his point of view, I suppose.

Talking about professional courtesy, this reminds me of another encounter with a physician, an experience that sort of epitomized the environment in which I practiced acupuncture in those days. I developed a little prostatic problem and went to see this urologist downtown. When I told him that I also do acupuncture, I could observe his eyes rolling back about 25 degrees before he forcibly stopped that action. Whether he was trying to teach me a lesson for straying off the mainstream of medicine, I don't know, but he gave me such a rough treatment in the examination room that in fact it became an unforgettable experience. He gave me a prostatic massage so vigorous that I almost threw-up. I could see a black curtain slowly draping down in front of me and I almost dropped to the floor. After this very powerful two-finger treatment from this gentleman, I suddenly realized being an acupuncturist was like being a heretic in the Spanish Inquisition. While professional courtesy was the standard practice in those days, he didn't give me any.

Fortunately, all of you will be practicing acupuncture in much more favorable environment.

Second point: There is an old Chinese saying, "If you believe everything the book says, it's better to be without the book." A book, no matter how good it is, is not going to tell you the whole truth and nothing but the truth. And you have to take everything with at least half a grain of salt.

Once upon a time, the dean of a very outstanding medical school addressed the graduating class on commencement day and said, "About 50% of what we taught you is going to be proven wrong. Unfortunately, we don't know which 50%." In this particular acupuncture course, you can be sure at least 80% of what we teach you is right, and we know which 80%. Like everything else, politics is always involved and acupuncture is no exception. Traditional Chinese medicine is no exception. It happens here in modern times, but also happened in China in ancient times. So if you think traditional Chinese medicine is a body of knowledge that is completely free of controversies, you'll be mistaken, because controversies always exist. Fortunately, the system of traditional Chinese medicine has been tested for so long and on so many people that some of the issues in dispute have been satisfactorily resolved.

So you'll encounter various different schools of thought, each emphasizing a certain aspect of traditional Chinese medicine. In a way, it is not unlike some of the development of religions. For example, in Christianity, you have the Baptists, Presbyterians, Lutherans, Roman Catholics, Anglicans, Eastern Orthodox and so on down the line. In Buddhism, you have the Red Sect, the Yellow Sect, the Zen and the like, and everybody will emphasize that their version of the truth is the only truth. And if you are not careful, you will fall into the trap of thinking that whatever knowledge in acupuncture you acquired is gospel. So my advice to you is to use your sense, use your reasoning power to dissect the teachings to see if it makes good sense to you.

Throughout the course you will have the opportunity to experience different styles of acupuncture, and you will hear diverse opinions about how things should be done from different faculty members. This is to allow you to have a wider range of contact with practitioners in the field. The emphasis in our course is on the concept of traditional Chinese medicine and how to integrate it into modern medicine.

As the third issue, some of you may say or ask, well I just want to treat patients with chronic pain; why do I need to know or learn about TCM or traditional Chinese medicine? My answer to you is that acupuncture is an integral part of traditional Chinese medicine. They are so interwoven that you cannot separate one from the other. If you just concentrate on acupuncture without any attention to the theory behind it or the use of herbal treatment, you're missing out on something. On the other hand, if you just simply use herbal treatment without any knowledge of the acupuncture system, the meridians or the acupuncture points, you also will not be as effective as you could be. That's why the most ancient formal text on traditional Chinese medicine is called "Yellow Emperor's Classic on Internal Medicine" or "Nei Jing" which translates to the Canon of Internal Medicine, which actually consists of two volumes. The first volume is called Ling Shu, the second volume Su Wen. Ling Shu means "wonderful hinges" as in door hinges, or "wonderful switches", because acupuncture points are like switches. They can switch on or switch off a certain function, just like you would open or close a door,. It is for this reason that a substantial volume of its text is devoted to the theory and practice of acupuncture. Whereas Su Wen which means "pure questioning", concentrates on the principles of medicine; it was written in a question and answer format. The questions of how to perform healing originated from the Yellow Emperor, Huang Di, who posited the questions to Qi Bo, who was the most prominent healer at the time.

Huang Di and Qi Bo lived in an era approximately 5000 years ago, whereas the Yellow Emperor's Classic on Internal Medicine, the book Nei Jing itself, was written around 400 BC. So the authors actually borrowed the names of Huang Di and Qi Bo to give the book a more authoritative appearance. It is worthwhile to note that as early as 2400 years ago, the system of traditional Chinese medicine was already highly developed and very sophisticated. As a matter of fact, even today we are still trying to understand some of the passages contained in this ancient text. Again, this book is living proof that acupuncture and medicine are so interconnected that you cannot really separate the two.

In modern medicine, the best way to combat a disease state is to understand the pathogenesis. Likewise, in Chinese medicine, one must know the causation of a certain medical condition before one can deal with it effectively.

According to the traditional Chinese medical principles, a blockage of the flow of the vital energy known as "qi" (pronounced "chee") will cause pain, as well as a whole host of other physical and mental symptoms. So if you want to determine the cause of the problem, you'll look into the symptom complex and then draw a conclusion as to why the patient is suffering from this particular set of problems, so that you can devise the way to overcome this blockage of qi or energy. Just like in modern days, if you were told that the major roadway leading to a certain city is blocked, you would want to find out the exact cause. Is it blocked because of a fallen tree? Is it blocked due to flooding? A mudslide? Knowing the exact cause, you will be able to find a solution to open up that roadway. For example, if it is a fallen tree, you would need to bring a big chainsaw; if it is a mudslide, then you'd better bring in the heavy equipment to move the earth. And if it is caused by a flood, then you'll probably have to bring in sandbags.

A parallel can be found in the human body. If there is a blockage of the flow of qi in a certain channel, it may be due to entrapment of heat or qi congestion. And the solution for that is to use acupuncture or other means to disperse the qi, to vent out the excessive energy, so to speak. On the other hand, if it is caused by wetness, or phlegm syndrome, then you may want to use moxibustion, using the herbal fragrance as well as the heat to warm up the system to get rid of the moisture. Yet if the cause is the so-called "blood clot syndrome", then you'll need to dissolve the clot by whatever means you have available. And since blood is often related to the liver-gallbladder meridian system, you may want to stimulate those systems to resolve this particular condition.

If the cause of this blockage of qi is qi deficiency, then what you need is to tonify the system, to give it more energy to replenish its energy. And if the condition is a result of excessive cold, then what you need to do is to use a warming treatment to try to bring up the activity of those systems.

Each of those causes manifests with its own other symptoms, but the common objective symptom of all these conditions is pain.

So pain is a symptom which may be caused by a multitude of problems. And how do you understand these problems? By studying the whole of traditional Chinese medicine, not just some parts.

Once you know how these different causes can lead to different symptom complexes, you can devise a way to reverse those problems. And if you restrict yourself in the treatment of pain only and ignore all the other symptoms, you are missing the point, literally. So even if your specialty is anesthesiology or physical rehabilitation, you need to know the patient in every which way. Now you'll be able to apply the principles of traditional Chinese medicine to allow you to more effectively handle the problems.

This whole exercise is like learning how to fish. If you are taught how to cast the line, how to put the bait on the hook, how to dress up in fishing gear, and how to wade into the river, you are getting only part of the training. You must know how to pick the spot where you can find a fish. You must know the season for fishing. You might want to find out what time of the day a fish would be looking for food. You should have some knowledge of the currents and the behavior of the fish you're trying to get. Without this knowledge, you will be able to catch some fish some of the time, but you won't be able to get most of the fish you could have gotten, most of the time.

And it is for this reason that we try to teach you not only how to find the points, where to put the needles for certain conditions, and the technique of inserting needles, but we'll try to provide you with the basic knowledge of how to analyze a clinical problem, and how to decide the treatment modality and treatment direction so you'll be able to maximize the therapeutic benefit for your patients.

Now, what if you ignore all these principles, and just go ahead and do a cookbook approach, a recipe approach? All right, if you have back pain, I am going to use these two points and those three points. If you have headaches, I'm going to use this set of points and I use it on everybody. Would you be able to help the patient? Yes, you would be able to help the patient. But you won't be able to help the patient as much as you can. Let's say you can help 50% of the patients and get them to improve 50% using the cookbook approach, a 50/50 proposition. You multiply that: .5 x .5 is .25, so your satisfaction score is .25. On the other hand, if you're able improve the clinical outcome by making 80% of your patients 80% better, what kind of satisfaction score do you get? .8 x .8 is .64. .64 is almost 3 times as good as .25. And imagine what this difference in efficacy can do for your practice. If your patients are three times more satisfied with your treatment, would these patients refer you their friends and relatives? Would their doctors refer you patients if they see this kind of result, instead of a .25 satisfactory score? You bet they will. It is easy to see that an improvement of the efficacy of your treatments would have a major impact on your practice.

Issue number four: You ask the question, if people go to school for traditional Chinese medicine for 3 or 4 years to become professional acupuncturists, how can I learn it in just a few hundred hours? In traditional Chinese medicine school in China, it is a 3 year program, this is true. But in that curriculum, the portion of time devoted to the teaching of acupuncture is quite a bit less than the total time spent on, say, the traditional Chinese medicine theories and herbal treatments. Here we aren't teaching you herbal medicine. We just basically teach you acupuncture, so the time is much more commensurable with the time spent on the subject of acupuncture in a traditional Chinese medicine school, and that's the first point. Now, you also should never, never underestimate your ability as a physician, because by this time you have already spent on the average perhaps 12 years learning medicine. You have seen critical conditions. You have seen dying patients. You have taken care of emergencies. These situations do not faze you because you lived that experience throughout your training, and that counts for a lot. In the old days, the traditional acupuncturists and herbalists saw all sorts of critical conditions – traumas, injuries, near death conditions, so they were very experienced. But in modern times, many herbalists do not have exposure to various serious conditions, especially outside of China. You have also learned all the basic sciences: You have learned anatomy, physiology, and you have a great understanding of how the body functions and how it is structured. So for you, it will be a lot simpler to learn acupuncture than somebody who is totally without training in these areas.

To illustrate my point, let me tell you a little story. During the late Ching Dynasty, there was a very famous martial artist named Hong Xi Guan. Hong was a graduate of the Shaolin temple. He was one of the most accomplished martial artists. During his travel to the south of China, he noticed a nun was practicing a most peculiar kung fu style, which was because the movements were imitative of those of the tiger and the crane. So he asked this nun to teach him the style. After finding out who he really was, the nun replied, "I can teach you but you must do something for me in return." Hong asked, "What do you want me to do?" The nun said, "I'm a nun; I cannot commit any act of violence against another human being, but before I became a nun my father was murdered by this criminal but I'm not able to avenge him, and I feel ashamed." Hong became the disciple of this nun, and in return he agreed to seek revenge for her. Hong was able to learn everything he had to learn from her in a matter of thirty days, which normally would have taken an ordinary person years to accomplish. He was able to learn this new style so quickly because he was already trained in martial arts. The foundation of learning had already been laid. By the way, Hung did avenge her father eventually.

Ladies and gentlemen, as a physician, you have all the training necessary to make you a fast learner of this healing art, so do not underestimate the value of training which may not appear to have a lot to do with acupuncture on the surface but in fact does, because the purpose of our learning is to heal others, and we have done that for years. Learning acupuncture is like learning how to swim. After basic swimming lessons you still won't be able to swim across the English Channel in wintertime without a wetsuit; that's too much to expect. But now you can swim across an Olympic size pool a number of laps, you know how to tread water, so if you are thrown into the ocean, you will not drown right away. You will be able to survive long enough to get on to a life raft, or to be rescued. These few hundred hours of training will not make you into a highly accomplished acupuncturist, but will at least give you a very, very sound starting point. You'll be amazed how much good you can do for your patients, even with these couple of hundred hours of training. But of course you have to assert yourself, you have to study hard, you have to put in the hours, and you have to practice; there are no two ways about it. And let me remind you that in China, the barefoot doctors did acupuncture on huge numbers of patients, and most of them did not even have a high school education. Yet they were able to help a lot of people with this technique, and that's the beauty of acupuncture.

You will see it is one of the safest procedures, if you follow certain specific guidelines. That's why I often say acupuncture is for the best doctors but is also for the worst doctors. For the best doctors, because you get to use this technique to do a lot of good for a lot of patients by applying your deductive power, your reasoning, your analytical ability, and so on and so forth, in any number of clinical situations, and that's why the technique is an excellent tool for the best doctors. On the other hand, it is so safe that even less competent doctors will be able to administer this treatment safely and relatively effectively. That's not to say that any of you is less than competent. I have full confidence that you're all well trained. but to illustrate the point, even less qualified individuals, such as the barefoot doctors, are not likely to do any harm if you give them proper training.

You must, however, follow certain rules in a very strict manner to avoid doing any harm to your patients, which we will teach you as the course develops. You have already been trained to handle a lot of needling techniques with big needles, to say the least. Naturally you are able to draw blood, give immunization shots, perhaps perform thoracocentesis, liver biopsy, arterial puncture, lumbar puncture and so on and so forth. So you have already a lot of experiences with needles under your belt; adding acupuncture to your therapeutic armamentarium should come pretty easy for you. Your attitude, if you should have one, is to be proud and humble at the same time. This is not a contradiction in terms. You're proud because you have good solid background in medicine. You should also be humble because there are always new things to be learned, new techniques to be acquired and new insights to be obtained.

The fifth philosophical point I want to make regarding this course is about integrating the east and the west. You must learn both the faults and the merits of both systems, and how to make the best of the combined approach. There's plenty that is right about modern medicine. It is extremely effective in treating trauma, although as time goes on, one must realize that traditional Chinese medicine has a lot to contribute also in this particular field. It's highly effective in treating infections, although the resistance to antibiotics is putting a cramp on the style of modern drug therapy. Again, TCM will have something to contribute in this arena, and we shall talk about it further along in the course. Surgical interventions, fantastic advances in the past half a century: We're able to do organ transplant. We're able to do a lot of miraculous procedures. Immunizations allow us to virtually get rid of smallpox, and put polio under very tight control, and avoid many unnecessary deaths due to infections, through the use of immunization.

Modern medicine is also very good for the treatment of certain chronic diseases like gout. It does not cure it, but it will put a tight lid on its activities because we understand some of the underlying biochemical abnormalities associated with this condition. We're also able to save many lives from myocardial infarction, we're able to decrease the death rate substantially, and last but not least, modern medicine has been able to categorize many, many different diseases, put them under different headings, giving them very detailed description as to the symptoms, physical findings, abnormal biochemical findings, as well as their causes. And this is by and large, lacking in the system of traditional Chinese medicine.

But we also have a whole bunch of problems affiliated with the practice of modern medicine. There are many diseases with no cure and no treatments. There are just way too many side-effects that are severe enough to be life threatening, and oftentimes, we use one drug to overcome the side-effects of another drug, only to give rise to its own side-effects. Many of these drugs are potentially extremely dangerous and often disabling, and for many, many conditions, the modern approach is not entirely effective, if not outright ineffective, as we shall see in many chronically painful conditions. Sure, you can take pain pills, but the suppression of pain is often incomplete and it does not cure the condition per se, it merely suppresses the symptoms, and that is the failing of modern medicine.

And for many degenerative conditions, what we're trying to do is to sort of break the falls of their ever downward spiraling degenerative changes. But we're not able to either stop the spiral altogether, let alone to reverse it. What we western medical doctors are doing is simply buying time.

In contrast, the elegance of TCM or traditional Chinese medicine is that it can often actually reverse the disease process. It can permanently improve or even cure some disease conditions, including some hypertensions, asthmatic conditions, chronic pain, chronic fatigue syndrome, and so on. Now, oftentimes we may not be able to do a complete job or cause a complete reversal of the symptoms of a degenerative disease, but it does often do enough to make a difference.

The pitfall of TCM is sometimes it does not differentiate between disease entities very well. For example, if we refer to a shoulder pain, the shoulder pain may be caused by adhesive capsulitis or it may be caused by tendonitis or it may be caused by bursitis, or other conditions, but TCM oftentimes does not make a clear-cut distinction of one entity from another. So if we can combine the understanding from the viewpoints of western medicine and eastern medicine, it will make for a very good mix to get the best of both worlds. By specifying the western diagnosis, we know how the disease behaves, and we can design the treatment using the TCM understanding and principles to correct that situation. So the major impetus of this course is to attempt to integrate the eastern and western approaches to healing. When we do integrate these two systems, we do not have just integrated medicine, but rather, we have a system of super medicine, which is going to do a lot of things that previously we could not imagine.

The last philosophical issue I want to mention to you is, avoid dogma, avoid academic arrogance. I don't like dogma at all. Dogma is a bitch — "dog ma" right? Dogma will only procreate more dogmas, and we don't want that. Dogma restricts your point of view and allows you only to have tunnel vision. Spell dogma in reverse, it's AMGOD, "am god". Because I am god, you must do what I tell you to do and that's how dogma works.

In modern medicine, there are many dogmas. One of the dogmas is that if it cannot be explained by modern medical science, it couldn't possibly happen. So if a patient tells you specific symptoms that are so strange and unexplainable by what we know, we blame the patient because it's all in the head; these symptoms are not real, they don't exist. They exist only in the imagination of the patient. Let me ask you a question, "How often are you not able to explain what the patients told you?" Are they all crazy? No.

There's also the dogma of the separation of the body and the mind, or the dogma of body-mind dichotomy. It was not until recently that the barrier between physical illness and psychiatric illness began to breakdown. These are some of the examples of the dogma of Western medicine.

Acupuncture has its own dogma too. There is a modern school of acupuncture that proclaims that all the body ailments stem from the misalignment of teeth. If you fix the teeth, pull out the amalgam, align the teeth correctly, your physical problems will disappear. Apparently this belief was already quite rampant during the early part of the 20th century. Frank Lloyd Wright, the famous architect, actually had all his teeth pulled out because one of the curators at Guggenheim Museum, which he designed, told him that his ailments all came from his teeth. Academic arrogance is another problem of modern acupuncture, because people think that we know so much about anatomy, physiology; why do we need to use the system of meridians.

Chapter Two – Facts and Fallacies on Acupuncture and Traditional Chinese Medicine

Do you know how many years of painstaking research the ancient scholars in China worked to find the system of meridians, and in fact how many great medical minds were involved in the development of this system? And it's such a waste to throw it away just like that. As a matter of fact, these were the inventors of acupuncture. So why are we just learning some portions of those teachings, and discarding the rest? There are those modern physicians or acupuncturists who believe the advent of modern medical sciences, including the study of the human body, detailed anatomical dissections, and the present physiological understanding of how the body functions, gives them the permission to ignore all the work that was done by previous giants in the field of medicine.

These ancient scholars may in fact have been much more knowledgeable than we are, because they saw the intricacies and the complexities of the inner workings of the body. And just because we cannot explain it in terms of modern science does not give us carte blanche to throw it away. It will be a terrible loss if we allow this to happen. The meridian concept is truly the distillation of the intellectual prowess of many of the great minds that ever lived.

I was asked once, "What is it like to do acupuncture without the help of the meridians?"

Well, my answer was that it's like going to a strange town without a roadmap. It's like going to sea without a compass. It is like trying to reach an itch on your foot, but doing it on the outside of the boot. It is like having a salad without dressing, or worse, having the dressing without the salad. It is like making love without ever reaching climax.

To do acupuncture without using the meridians is to miss the key element of this healing art, so our attitude towards the principles and theories of acupuncture should be that if we cannot explain them readily with modern medical knowledge, we should at least preserve the concept. Put it on the back burner, if you will, and revisit them when we have more scientific data.

Now that we have visited the philosophical issues, maybe we should take a look at the whole body of knowledge of acupuncture itself.

What I say to you is that if you have some prior knowledge about acupuncture, that's good, and if you have no knowledge whatsoever, that's even better, because some of your preconceived notions may be quite wrong. A number of fallacies have prevailed in the public mind regarding acupuncture. Although acupuncture is now gaining wider acceptance among the public as well as the American medical community, it is still grossly underutilized in many clinical applications.

This is so because traditional theories on which acupuncture is based have been difficult to interpret in light of modern science. Modern western physicians find it hard to swallow the cocktail of acupuncture theory containing, say, one part of yin, not gin, one part of yang, a handful of meridians, a dash of qi, and a twist of five elements. As a logical foundation of acupuncture, these theories are considered unscientific at best, and superstitious at worst, since it is impossible for them to relate such seemingly metaphysical concepts directly to their real life experience. Worse yet, the lack of understanding of traditional Chinese medicine is far surpassed by the misunderstanding of it. To point out the seriousness and extent of such gross misunderstandings of this ancient but highly useful science of healing, let's examine some of the commonly held myths and fallacies about acupuncture.

Fallacy 1 – The theory of acupuncture is based on philosophy.

Well, for some most strange reason, many articles on acupuncture written by physicians as well as by non-physicians describe acupuncture as an ancient Chinese art of healing based on Taoist philosophy. No doubt, there was yin, yang, five elements, nature, etc., all of which do play roles in the themes of Taoist philosophy.

But to equate acupuncture with Taoism or philosophy per se is absolutely inaccurate. Historically speaking, there were ten prevailing schools of thought during the Chinese so-called Spring-Autumn Warring States period, which was between about 770 BC to 222 BC. The yin-yang theory is one such school. It explains the order of the universe in terms of two opposing vital forces in nature, called yin and yang. These theories belonged to a school of philosophy distinctly separate from Taoism and the eight other schools, including the well-known Confucianism. Taoism was, of course, founded by Lao Zhi. But keep in mind that long before the yin-yang proponents flourished, the concept of yin and yang was firmly embodied in the comprehensive system of traditional Chinese medicine, of which acupuncture was an integral part.

According to this concept, good health is a result of the harmonious interaction between the living organism, man himself, and his environment, that is, nature, and the maintenance within himself of a dynamic equilibrium of the vital forces known as yin and yang. This equilibrium, the harmonious internal state, what we know in modern times as the "milieu interior", had to a large extent influenced the thinking of the yin-yang proponents and the Taoists. Such a scientific principle or medical concept can have, of course, philosophical overtones, as many great discoveries in science often do. For example, Darwin's theory of evolution which bred the so-called "social Darwinism", was a sort of philosophy at the time. Obviously, to claim that the theory of evolution is a derivative of the social concept of survival of the fittest, is to put the cart before the horse. Similarly, it is equally preposterous to claim acupuncture or Chinese medicine for that matter, to be an offspring of any philosophy, let alone Taoism.

Acupuncture is a highly logical system of healing based on astute scientific observations accumulated throughout centuries, if not millennia. To incorrectly identify Chinese medical theories as a philosophy instead of a science helps only to arouse skepticism in the minds of modern western physicians. A contributory factor for such mistaken identity is the acupuncture lingo itself. Words such as yin, yang, five elements, wind, cold, fire, wetness, etc. naturally give acupuncture a very unscientific appearance, particularly to the western physicians who do not know what kind of physiological or the pathological processes they represent.

14

Nevertheless, if we do not insist on the exclusive use of modern technical terminology, but instead accept these terms as mere symbols which stand for definite physiological phenomena and clinical events, there need not be any more confusion. For example and for argument's sake, if the terms "sympathetic" and "parasympathetic" are substituted for "yin" and "yang" respectively -- well, these are approximations, not exact equivalents -- the mystery of these two unfamiliar words would then be dispelled instantly. And if we use "alpha, beta, gamma, omega and epsilon" to substitute for the five elements, namely metal, wood, water, fire, and earth, which in reality represent cycles of excitation and inhibition in the central nervous system -- or the relationships of the positive and negative feedback pathways among different physiological systems -- then acupuncture will take on a new look. It will even take on the cloak of scientific respectability. The situation is rather similar to a form of advanced mathematics known as topology, where terms like trees and grass are used. But to call topology horticulture just because these borrowed terms were used is simply ludicrous. Similarly, to call the theory of acupuncture a philosophy just because it contains words that have metaphysical overtones is equally preposterous.

Fallacy 2 – Acupuncture and Chinese medicine are folk medicine.

Acupuncture and Chinese medicine are not folk medicine. Although acupuncture has been viewed as an entity distinctly different from other methods of healing, it cannot be separated from the mainstream of traditional Chinese medicine, which also employs herbs of various sorts, since both forms of therapy are based on the same physiological concepts and therapeutic principles. To learn acupuncture without referring to the total system of TCM or traditional Chinese medicine, is much like learning surgery without the fundamental training in the basic sciences, or knowledge of the other disciplines of modern medicine. But most westerners, doctors and laymen alike, think of traditional Chinese medicine and by association acupuncture, as a form of folk medicine. This misinformation, gross as it may be, is quite understandable. In the awareness of most industrialized nations of the western world, modern medicine is the only legitimate means of treating illnesses, and in the experience of westerners, herbs are commonly used medically in the more primitive cultures, and their use is based on irregular empiricism. To them, Chinese medicine is not much more than some sort of ancient folk medicine, since it also uses herbs extensively as therapeutic agents. By labeling Chinese medicine as Chinese folk medicine, it immediately depreciates its value. As a result, physicians think to themselves, why should they expend their energy and effort to understand the trivialities of Chinese folk medicine.

Now of course, everybody is talking about herbs, talking about St. John's Wort, Gingko Biloba, Saw Palmetto, etc., etc. And most people, physicians included, think that Chinese herbal treatment is very similar to the, say, Native American herbal treatments, or other treatments with herbs. It is true that herbs are extensively used in TCM, but here is where the similarity between Chinese medicine and folk medicine ends. In fact, the term "Chinese herbal medicine" is a misnomer: In addition to medicinal plants, a wide variety of animal products, such as a toad skin which contains epinephrine, seal's testes, which contains testosterone, and minerals such as arsenic and mercury, are also used as therapeutic agents. Therefore it is a mistake to call traditional Chinese medicine herbal medicine simply because herbs are used, just as it is wrong to call modern western medicine western herbal medicine, with its use of digitalis, heparin, morphine, curare, oil of wintergreen, and so on, all of which happen to be plant derivatives. Quite unlike folk medicine, the pharmacological characteristics, therapeutic dosages and interactions of all these agents used in TCM had been carefully documented and reviewed in the Chinese medical literature throughout history. As a matter of fact, the imperial governments of various dynasties took an active interest in the preservation of this art of healing by constantly revising the "Ben Cao" which means herbology, a Chinese pharmacological encyclopedia, so to speak. Governmental agencies were even established to test the skills of physicians, and officials were designated to oversee medically related activities, sort of like the NIH or CDC of ancient China. Not only that, but generations of highly accomplished physicians contributed many, many volumes to the literature of Chinese medicine so all the techniques, all the methods, all the pharmacological uses of different plants and animal products have been very meticulously documented in volumes and volumes of books and manuscripts, and the practice of TCM and acupuncture have been experienced by generations and millions of citizens.

Unlike folk medicine, which tends to treat a limited number of ailments with limited means, and is founded on fragmented information and knowledge, traditional Chinese medicine utilizes a comprehensive, deductive and highly logical system, not only for therapy, but for definite diagnosis and prognosis as well. A comprehensive system of therapy as such is basically absent in all other forms of folk medicine.

Folk medicine is generally empirical. Chinese medicine including acupuncture is not. The stage of empiricism had long passed, even at the time the Yellow Emperor's Classic on Internal Medicine was published, which was around the 4th century BC, by which time this system of diagnosis and treatment was clearly established, and many of the therapeutic principles were well founded. Medicine was not prescribed and needles were not inserted until a clear diagnosis was made. This was accomplished by the taking of patient's history, and a physical examination consisting of observation of the patient's color, aura, the taking of the pulses, inspecting the tongue, feeling for painful spots on the body, etc.

It is in fact quite amazing, because the principles are quite similar to those of modern medicine. History taking not only concerns the present illness, but also social and emotional history, as well as a review of systems focusing on physical functions such as sleep, urination, defecation, sweating, eating, etc. The physical examination according to TCM also includes inspection of the body, palpation of the body, ascertaining points of hyperesthesia, observation of psychomotor activities, and the emotional state of the patient, in addition to the more commonly known diagnostic techniques. Only after this type of painstaking collection and analysis of clinical data can a practitioner of TCM determine the process of pathogenesis, and only then will a therapeutic regimen to counteract the underlying condition be designed. The entire treatment process is highly deductive and analytical so that the element of empiricism is kept at a minimum. We know in modern medicine we use a lot of so-called "pattern recognition", and then we'll prescribe medication for that condition. In traditional Chinese medicine, such pattern recognition is less important because most of the conclusions are reached by logical deduction, rather than fitting the pattern to a specific disease.

Fallacy 3 – What is unexplainable about acupuncture is also unacceptable.

Now, the traditional theory of acupuncture really revolves around such concepts as the interplay of the two vital forces known as yin and yang, the flow of qi in the meridians, the suppression and creation cycles of the five elements, and some other abstract notions that have so far completely defied modern scientific explanation.

However, to regard all unexplainable phenomena as invalid is really highly presumptuous because it is assumed that the present knowledge about the human body is both accurate and complete, and any other findings which are in direct conflict with such knowledge must be excluded. But of course, our present day knowledge within the western system of medicine is neither complete nor absolutely accurate. What we consider advanced scientific knowledge today may in fact be proven to be rather primitive tomorrow. Simply look at the ways diabetics have been advised in the past decades regarding their diet, and post-menopausal and pre-menopausal women about hormonal replacement therapy, both of which have been vacillating and fluctuating back and forth from time to time. First we said carbohydrates are bad, then we said carbohydrates are really good, that you don't have to restrict carbohydrates, and then we say now that fast absorbing carbohydrates are really not that good. And as far as hormonal replacement therapy goes, some days we say estrogen is good. On other days we say estrogen must be accompanied by progestin. And then we'll also say if you take the hormones, you may increase the chance of thromboembolic events. It can protect your bones, but you also increase the chance of having breast cancers, and so on.

So looking at this history, one must conclude that whichever doctors are giving out this advice must be running for political office. As these opinions seem to change with the wind, a number of well known figures in western medicine do not want to recognize the merit of acupuncture on its own. Many even refuse to acknowledge that acupuncture anesthesia actually works, and they'd rather attribute its efficacy to hypnosis and suggestion. Dr. Michael DeBakey, the famed cardiovascular surgeon, and Patrick Wall, the co-proponent of the gate control theory are among them. The main difficulty for modern physicians to accept acupuncture wholeheartedly is caused in part by their unwillingness to either entertain the idea or recognize the possibility that a healing art of such remote origin may embody some concepts and practices more advanced than those of modern medicine.

Let's examine how it is possible that a healing art of such ancient origin could embody some very advanced concepts. From a historical point of view, scientific achievements generally do not develop in parallel in different isolated societies; clearly, at one historical moment, society A may be far more advanced than society B, and sometime later the opposite may be true. So when Marco Polo first visited China in the 13th century, he found wonders by the dozens. He probably took back chow mein to Italy and called it spaghetti, and imported wonton and called it ravioli. But just only a few hundred years later, China was overwhelmed by the firearms, battleships, and other technological advances of the European nations, the products of the industrial revolution. If we follow the uneven development of human knowledge, then the knowledge of medicine might also have developed in very similar, uneven patterns in the East and the West. For example, in the 4th century BC, the system of Chinese medicine was already highly developed, and had already accumulated a few thousand years of medical experiences. Conversely, the bulk of advances in western medicine were made only in the last few hundred years. Western medicine focuses on the analysis of the body to as far as the molecular level, while Chinese medicine attempts to relate the various bodily functions and their interactions with one another, as well as with the environment. Ironically, this approach might not even have been possible, had it not been free from the bias of modern medicine. So, independently and without being influenced by each other, each focusing on a different aspect of the organism in health and disease, TCM and western medicine separately reached the present stage of development.

The theory of Chinese medicine is derived from the observation of the physiological manifestations basically of the central nervous system, whereas modern medicine long ignored the central nervous system in pathogenesis until recently. Unfortunately, since the central nervous system or CNS is the least understood part of the body in modern medicine, there's little wonder that much of the acupuncture phenomena remain inexplicable.

When we examine the ancient literature of TCM, we are surprised and in fact, amazed to find numerous examples of very advanced medical thinking. For example, it is maintained in the early book of medicine, the Nei Jing, that when the intake of salt is excessive, the pulse hardens, which is really the rationale of current therapy of hypertension with diuretics. This passage in that book established a clear connection between the intake of salt and hypertension. In another example: It's well known now in the western world that Harvey discovered circulation a few hundred years ago but it remains obscure even to most Chinese that as early as more than two millennia ago, the Nei Jing already stated that the heart is the master of blood and that blood flows along vessels to irrigate and nourish the whole body, essentially reaching the same conclusion as Harvey did some 2000 years later. In recent years despite the lack of satisfactory modern scientific interpretation of the bulk of the traditional Chinese medical theories, many clinical applications have been conducted following these ancient principles in the People's Republic of China, with outstanding results.

Diseases such as bronchial asthma and anovulatory functional uterine bleeding, lupus erythematous and certain neurasthenia, that are generally thought to be distinct pathological entities by modern medicine, were noted to share a number of constitutional symptoms, which according to traditional theories, are associated with a so-called deficient kidney system or kidney qi deficiency, which we'll discuss in some detail later on. So according to TCM, the kidney system probably represents not only the urogenital system, but also the autonomic system, the adrenal, and certain CNS functions. On the practical level, therapy with Chinese medical agents or herbal agents using the guidelines of these traditional theories yielded remarkable results. The therapeutic response was also accompanied by objective changes in the patterns of, say, the 24 hour urinary excretion of 17-hydroxy and 17 ketocortico steroids. The treatment of fractures with Chinese therapeutic agents combined with flexible splints instead of the modern conventional immobile casts is still another area of clinical triumph, resulting from the direct application of traditional medical principles.

Among many other successes is, of course, the shining example of acupuncture analgesia, on which we'll also spend just a little time trying to elucidate its mechanism.

Only very recently, modern physicians of the West began to realize the vital roles of emotional stresses in causing diseases. In recent decades, there has been a movement of holistic medicine trying to deal with health at the level of the body, mind and spirit. But you know what? The ancient Chinese physicians not only recognized this close relationship between psyche and soma, but also went further, to point out specifically what type of emotional excess causes what kind of physical illness, by correlating each emotion with its specific internal organ system. For instance, fear is associated with the kidney system, sorrow with the lung, anger with the liver, etc.

The demise of two of the world's richest men illustrates these Chinese medical principles. Howard Hughes suffered from excessive fear of germs while he was dying from chronic renal failure. He hid himself in a room, afraid to touch anything, and his favorite diet was Campbell's soup, using its high salt content to keep on stimulating his kidney system. Aristotle Onassis developed myasthenia gravis shortly after his only son's sudden death in a plane crash. According to TCM, the psychic stress of extreme longing after losing someone dear adversely affects the muscular system of the body. Modern medical research has implicated the central nervous system as the site of pathogenesis in a variety of disorders. The irreversible shock syndrome, neurogenic factors in both renal and essential hypertensions, the type A personality in association with coronary heart disease, stress ulcers, etc…etc… all involve the CNS. Acupuncture cures diseases by directly modulating central nervous system functions, so it is not surprising that it can treat such a wide spectrum of diseases. We should only be surprised at the very fact that we have ignored the CNS for so long, and call every symptom psychogenic if we cannot explain it from what we learned in medical school.

With such a vast body of evidence, the argument against acceptance of TCM is flimsy indeed, especially when we use so many drugs in modern medicine, about whose modes of action we understand little, and persist in employing surgical procedures with yet unproven value. So why should we treat TCM, acupuncture or other forms of alternative medicine with such a double standard?

Fallacy 4 – In order to prove that acupuncture really works, research must be done, using double-blind randomized control studies at university medical centers.

Recently when a hot-shot orthopedic department chairman of a major university medical school went to China and visited Beijing Hospital, he saw floors and floors of patients being treated by acupuncture for various medical problems. So he approached his counterpart, the Chinese professor, and said to him, "You know you've got so many patients with a similar diagnosis; this is a perfect environment to do double-blind control studies." The Chinese professor paused for a moment and then gently replied, "When the patient comes in, we know exactly what floor to send him to." What was left unsaid by the Chinese professor is that, well, we know it works. Acupuncture works, and if you want to prove to your own satisfaction that acupuncture really works, be my guest - do the double-blind control study. But we don't need that. Why waste time?

Do you think this technique of treatment would have survived if it hadn't worked for the last several thousand years, over vast territories of China, with millions and millions and millions of patients? Indeed, what the Chinese professor should have said is that quite a number of control studies were carried out as early as the 1950s. For instance, acupuncture was employed to treat infectious hepatitis and mumps. Both the course of the disease and the duration of the individual symptoms were much shortened in the treatment group, compared to the control group. The impression that the western physicians got, that not many disease conditions have been subjected to control study, because carefully controlled studies of acupuncture probably have not been carried out for every disease entity, is simply not true. The Chinese have long passed the stage of asking the question of whether acupuncture works. Instead, the most important question now is why and how it works, how it can be made to work better, and a great number of very important animal experiments on acupuncture have been carried out in China recently to that end. As a matter of fact, many of the investigative research works on clinical acupuncture done at certain university medical centers are really redundant efforts to prove what has already been proven.

If you look at the American literature, you'll find that there has been quite a bit of conflicting results in using acupuncture for control studies. Currently, one of the most popular ways of designing studies is to use what is known as sham acupuncture -- in other words, needles are inserted in places that are not acupuncture points -- and compare the result of these sham experiments with real acupuncture, where needles are inserted at actual acupuncture points themselves. Unfortunately, some of the western investigators themselves are not very well trained in acupuncture; they just know where the point is anatomically. When they inserted the needles, they paid no attention to how deep the needles should have gone, or whether that *de qi* phenomenon was obtained. What is the *de qi* phenomenon? When you insert the needle, you are supposed to "get the qi", or a response from the point as if the needle has been grabbed from underneath and tugged on a little bit, and with it, the patient experiences a special sensation traveling along a pathway with radiation of numbness, of tingling, of congestion, and so on and so forth. Without that kind of response, the treatment is usually ineffective because the needle is not necessarily in the acupuncture point itself. So when someone is not proficient in doing acupuncture, he is actually performing sham acupuncture unintentionally, when he was trying to do regular, real acupuncture.

On the other hand, acupuncture points are all over the body, and sometimes when they selected the so-called sham points, they were actually really good acupuncture points. So the points may actually be effective in treating that particular condition that was the subject of the research. The intent of the clinical trial was to compare the results between the control group using "sham acupuncture" and the experimental group using real acupuncture. In reality, however, because the techniques were used incorrectly, real acupuncture could be sham acupuncture and sham acupuncture may be real acupuncture. So the difference in outcome is greatly minimized between the two groups, and then they proclaim, "Well, there is no statistical difference between the two groups, and therefore, acupuncture is not effective."

The second problem associated with this kind of research is what I call "the one size fits all problem". When you go to a department store or a clothing store, you want to buy a jacket or a blouse. Because of your physique -- you may be tall, may be short, may be a little bit plump, may be a little bit skinny -- you want to pick out the size that fits you. Likewise, an acupuncture treatment, must be tailored to the individual patient, in order to make it work. So if you use the same protocol, exactly the same combination of points on different patients, their response, even though the official diagnosis is the same, may be utterly different. So, when you do research, you're not really allowed to deviate from the protocol, and you're going to use the same combination of points and the same techniques on every single patient, though they may have different constitutions and symptomatology, or causes of their conditions may vary according to TCM. So the therapeutic response may be uneven. And in real life, acupuncture treatments may need to be changed from time to time because the disease process is a dynamic one; it's ever-changing; it's evolving at all times. So you must tailor-make the treatments for that patient according to the responses you have gotten from the previous treatment. It is really not unlike the playing of a chess game. Your opponent is the disease process and you're playing against it. After you stimulate certain acupuncture points, the disease process changes, as if it has made a countermove. So depending on what countermove it has made, you have to make the next move to counter that, in order to win the match. So the dynamics of acupuncture treatments -- and the dynamics of the evolution of the condition -- have not been taken into account in the design of acupuncture treatment protocol for this type of research. And because you are not allowed to change your approach according to the response, you may not be able to effectively render the treatment. So the treatment results are not as good. In this case your conclusion will be warped because that particular treatment may not be fully effective for that particular medical condition.

For instance, different kinds of elbow pain may have different etiologies according to traditional Chinese medicine. So using the same formula approach to treat elbow pain may have an uneven response, depending on what condition one might have. Whereas if you tailor the treatment according to the individual condition, you may be able to achieve 80% improvement, but if you just use the one single protocol approach, you may be able to achieve only 40% improvement. Therefore, the conclusion based on this kind of single protocol for elbow pain would only show a moderate, instead of marked improvement of the condition. The clinical researchers in the ivory tower of the academic institutions such as major university medical schools will almost always insist on the double-blind randomized control study format, otherwise, any research done any other ways will not be completely satisfactory. While I agree that the double-blind control study model is an excellent one for many clinical situations, that is not the only way to accomplish the truth-finding mission.

Just ponder this for a moment: If Einstein and Darwin had been forced to do experiments to prove their points, they would have never been able to accomplish what they did, because neither of them did a single experiment. In the first case, Einstein did all the thinking, but no experiments. He made multiple observations of the physical world and then used his deductive power to finalize his theory of relativity. Darwin, on the other hand, travelled on board the ship Bugle, observing various kinds of creatures all over the world and came to the startling conclusion that all living things originated from a common ancestor, and various species are a result of a process called evolution. He too, used his power of observation and deduction to come up with the earthshaking theory of evolution. Acupuncture and the entire system of traditional Chinese medicine probably came about from a collection of very astute observations of how diseases developed and how treatments actually worked, culminating in a very complete and comprehensive system of medicine. I am by no means downgrading the importance of double-blind control studies. These are very, very helpful in many clinical situations, especially when the therapy takes a long time to manifest its effects and the effects may be more subtle, so the use of controls and placebos will document by comparison how effective the treatment really is.

To illustrate my point, just consider the following situation. If you were to get up out of your chair and walk out of the room though the door, where I put a big block of wood which you call a stumbling block, you would trip. So you would immediately conclude that the block made you trip and fall, and I come to you and say, "No, no, no, no. Your conclusion may not be valid because we really cannot be sure whether it is the physical existence of the block, or just the sight of the block that caused you to lose your balance and fall." So in order to really isolate the effects, we really need to do a sham stumbling block experiment. We'll put a block of the exact same size at the door, but this is not a real block, it's just a hologram created by lasers, and now you walk through the door. If you don't stumble, then we can conclude that the block itself is really the cause of your fall.

I am sure you agree that it is totally unnecessary to do this experiment. Why? Because you can associate the cause and effect very quickly; it is just common sense. So let me suggest to you that in many clinical situations, the therapeutic efficacy of acupuncture can be observed quickly and dramatically, so that you cannot be confused between the cause and the effect.

Let me also give you an example: At one time a patient was referred to me by an orthopedic surgeon. The patient had chronic low back pain for more than 5 years and after the first acupuncture treatment, the next day he felt 80% better and that improvement sustained for the next several days. When I saw him for the second time, I gave him an additional treatment and this time he was 90% better. Altogether I gave him three treatments, and his longstanding pain of more than five years disappeared totally. After thanking me for relieving his chronic malady, he actually complained to his orthopedic surgeon. He said, "Why didn't you refer me to Dr. Lee so I wouldn't have had to suffer for the last five years?" Of course, the orthopedic surgeon told him that "I haven't known Dr. Lee for five years. I just met him; that's why I referred you to him."

In another example, a disabled sheriff had had coronary bypass surgery three or four years earlier, in his early 40s. Subsequent to the operation, he developed chest pain that seemed to emanate from the thoracotomy scar. Since I had never treated a case like this before, I told the patient that I could only try to help him to relieve his pain that had been bothering him for a few years and was quite severe. To my surprise and to his astonishment, after one single treatment, the pain was almost entirely gone. He just couldn't believe it. Well, I'm sure somebody will say, this is anecdotal; maybe the patient was going to get well anyway. But what do you estimate the chances are, that someone suffering from a chronic severe pain for a number of years would suddenly get well literally overnight, after one single acupuncture treatment? What is the probability that it would happen as a random event? That possibility is extremely remote statistically.

Keep in mind that in ancient times, the Chinese did not conduct any double-blind studies, and the patients were mostly farmers, not necessarily well educated or sophisticated.

And they couldn't wait around to get better, because if they stopped working, they would not be able to bring in any income for their families. And the practice of acupuncture could be sustained for century after century because it worked, and worked quickly most of the time. And the therapeutic result is often dramatic and clear cut, so that you really have to be triple-blind not to see it. Despite the fact that acupuncture is getting more popular than ever, in my view, it is not quite popular enough. Because many of your colleagues particularly right in the mainstream will still say that acupuncture is unproven in its efficacy. And you need to make arguments in defense of the practice of acupuncture.

One of the arguments will be that many of the actual procedures done in modern medicine are equally unproven. They were not substantiated by double-blind control studies at all. If the same rigor were to apply to those procedures as are applied to acupuncture, then we should seriously question the validity of coronary bypass procedures themselves. So, following the same line of reasoning of those advocating sham acupuncture for clinical acupuncture research, sham operations should be done for all those patients undergoing coronary bypass surgeries.

The sham operation shall consist of opening up the chest, but without actually doing the grafting. Only in this way can we be sure that the effect of the bypass surgery is due to the grafting of the bypassed vessels, and not due to just the cutting open of the chest wall. Because there have been reports where, when the chest was opened in attempt to do the surgery, but without surgery itself actually done, the patient in fact felt better as a result of this operation without the actual graft. This is actually not as unreasonable a request as it seems; as we shall see later, by injecting points on the chest wall or trigger points on the chest wall, oftentimes anginal pain can be relieved or even pain with acute myocardial infarction. And in China, making an incision at an acupuncture point to treat various medical conditions has been tried, and often with much longer lasting results than just using the acupuncture needles alone. Yet, thousands and thousands of patients have undergone bypass surgeries at a cost of billions of dollars, where sham operations have never been done to prove once and for all that the coronary bypass surgery itself does, in fact, benefit patients.

Similarly, brain surgery has been employed to treat Parkinson's disease, but is there a possibility that just opening the skull has a curative effect? Because we know for a fact that by using scalp acupuncture, one can actually affect the motor disorders of many patients, including Parkinson's disease, by stimulating the scalp which overlies the area of the motor cortex in the brain. So by just inserting needles and stimulating that area on the scalp, the practitioner can induce some positive effects in the body, counteracting some of the symptoms relating to the motor cortex and the extrapyramidal system. Then the incision itself on the scalp, and even more so, the cutting open of the skull, or craniotomy, should have an even more dramatic effect. It is my understanding that Johns Hopkins University is actually toying with this idea of doing a sham craniotomy, compared to the real operation, to see if there is any difference in the therapeutic outcome. In fact, the protocol as I understand has already passed the committee on human experimentation.

Now let's take a look at another reason so often quoted by non-believers of acupuncture. They'll say, "Well, sure acupuncture works, but it works not because of its physiological effect, but rather due to the placebo effect. Patient perceives something is being done for them and therefore they're hopeful and somehow they get better." This view is in fact held by some famous pain researchers that I personally know.

To counter this argument, let's take a look at placebo effects. Think of placebo as a drug, and as a drug, we can analyze the pharmacokinetics of this drug. One should really study the placebo effects in great detail. For example, what is its absorption rate? In other words, how long does it take for the placebo effect to be apparent? One hour, one day, one week? And then we should also ask the question: What is its duration of action? Does the placebo effect work indefinitely, or will it just wane after a while? Does it have a half-life? Say, after one week its effect is only 50% of the effect first perceived? How long should it be expected to last? And what is its percentage of effectiveness?

In other words, if you randomly give the placebo to a patient population, in what percentage of these patients should you expect to see some effect of the placebo? Does a pill we call placebo interact with other agents, therapeutic or otherwise? For instance, if you send a bill collecting agent to talk to the patients, will the placebo effect disappear instantly? As they may tell you that they have never gotten better. Is there something called negative placebo effect, in which case, after the acupuncture treatment or sham acupuncture treatments, they actually feel worse? What percentage of the patient population actually develops this anti-placebo effect? Do we also expect sham placebo to be different from the real placebo? In real acupuncture the needle is inserted more deeply; in sham acupuncture, the needle is only touching the skin, or barely goes through the very superficial areas of the body. So, would there be a different degree of placebo effect?

What I'm suggesting here is to establish all the parameters of the placebo effect, so that they may be subtracted from the observed effect.

Let's say, given a population of 100 patients, 60 of them improved for more than 10 days from a single treatment. And if we know that by all experimentation and all studies, the placebo effect is only effective in 1/3 of the patient population, and if its effect does not last, say, more than 2 days, then we know in this particular situation, the additional 30% or so of patients in this group has experienced something much more than the placebo, and the therapeutic effect lasting such a long time is not accountable by using the placebo concept alone, because the observed clinical improvement far exceeded the best placebo effect one can obtain.

Therefore, if the clinical improvement cannot be explained by placebo effect, then acupuncture must be doing something positive for the patient population. Using this placebo subtraction process, we can actually avoid doing the sham acupuncture by simply having a control versus the treatment group. The control group is still necessary, because there are additional factors other than placebo, such as the environment, the changing of the weather, the changing of the barometric pressure, all of which may affect the clinical course or the symptoms, and as we shall see later, the fluctuation of the biorhythm or the body's basal energy level, which can lead to both clinical improvement and clinical deterioration. And these apparent effects must be subtracted from the real effects.

Finally, the university setting may not be the only proper setting in which good acupuncture research can be done. Many scientific breakthroughs actually have sprung from serendipity, not planned research. The spark of research ideas often arises from the practice of the art itself. The strides made in China during recent years in the field of acupuncture are really a direct result of the pulling of practical experience from a large number of practitioners. Indeed, non-research activities in acupuncture are needed to fuel the engine of research. Therefore, ladies and gentlemen, you have a vital role to play.

Finally, Fallacy 5 -- Acupuncture may be effective for Chinese people, but not necessarily for Americans, due to cultural differences.

Well, American physicians in general express a varying degree of skepticism about the efficacy of acupuncture. Even those who accept the fact that acupuncture analgesia works well in China have doubts about its efficacy on Americans. Stoicism as a result of indoctrination, has been the most commonly cited reason for the ability of thousands of Chinese men, women and children to undergo operations in the wakeful state, and without apparent distress, using acupuncture as the only form of analgesia. Americans, they have explained, are not culturally conditioned to tolerate pain, and therefore may not be susceptible to acupuncture analgesia. Speculation of this sort implies there is no neurophysiological basis for acupuncture analgesia, only a psychological one. Patrick Wall of England, the co-proponent of the gate control theory, went so far as to regard acupuncture analgesia as a matter of distraction. However, the body of evidence now available weighs heavily against this kind of explanation. For example, one would be hard-pressed to explain why acupuncture analgesia works on animals, as they certainly are not noted for their stoicism, nor have they received cultural conditioning of any kind. More importantly, these spokesmen have overemphasized acupuncture analgesia, and ignored the fact that acupuncture was developed several millennia ago, and has since been used to treat a wide spectrum of disorders, not just for killing pain. Psychological factors cannot possibly account for the successful use of acupuncture in resuscitation or for the control of asthmatic conditions.

So many dynasties came and left, governments were established and then overthrown, while acupuncture is still alive and well. It is unthinkable that acupuncture could have survived so long without being a highly effective modality of treatment, particularly in view of the immense cultural changes throughout the history of China.

Chapter Three – Yin and Yang of Nature and Nature of Yin and Yang

We have touched upon the physiological approach to the learning of acupuncture. Let's take a look of the basic concepts of traditional Chinese medicine. It is very, very important to know the concepts, because without the concepts, you will be lost. And it is difficult to achieve greatness without the building blocks of this knowledge. Can you learn acupuncture without having to learn these concepts first? The answer is yes, of course, because the barefoot doctors in China did not necessarily have to learn all the theories of traditional Chinese medicine, yet they were able to dispense or prescribe treatment for a large number of people in their community. Let's use a simple analogy. A doctor is like an auto mechanic, although the auto mechanic may sometimes disagree, because I remember one time I told an auto mechanic he was just like a doctor. He said, "No, don't compare me with a doctor. I know what I am doing."

So if you use the cookbook approach or the recipe approach, you may be able to use one set of points to treat, say, allergic rhinitis, and another set of points to treat low back pain. You would be able to do some good for your patients. However, you would not be able to maximize therapeutic efficacy for the more complicated cases. You'd be more like the assistant auto mechanic or the helper to the mechanic. You may be able to change some spark plugs, you may be able to change some tires, you may be able to fix some simpler problems, but you'll never be the chief auto mechanic.

But what we are trying to achieve here is more than turning you into an auto mechanic or even a chief auto mechanic. We want you to have the potential to become an automotive engineer or even the innovative mechanical engineer who develops a more efficient engine that will have great fuel economy, up to 80 miles per gallon of gasoline, and with the know-how to invent an electric car which will be able to eliminate air pollution altogether. And in order to do so, you must learn all the basics, such as physics and math. The equivalent of physics and math in acupuncture are the concepts of traditional Chinese medicine.

Let's now begin the discussion on the concept of yin and yang, which is perhaps the single most important concept in the entire body of knowledge in traditional Chinese medicine. In a prior meeting with physicians, I asked the participants what are the definitions of yin and yang, and I got a whole bunch of different answers. Some said they are male and female, others said they are positive and negative, but few understood the true meaning of the words yin and yang.

So let's backtrack a minute and to see if there's a simple way of explaining this fundamental concept. In Chinese, the word yang means the sun, and yin means the shade or the absence of sun, and all other characteristics of yin and yang are really derivatives of this simple concept. So daytime, when the sun is present, is the yang part of the 24-hour daily cycle, while night, during the absence of the sun, is the yin component of the cycle.

In the presence of the sun there is plenty of light, so light is yang, whereas the absence of light or darkness is yin. You have to look up in the sky to see the sun, so the upward direction is yang. And when you look away from the sun, you look downward, so the downward direction is yin. The sun radiates not only light but heat, so a high temperature is considered to be yang, whereas a low temperature is considered to be yin.

This has, of course, actual applications in clinical situations regarding the patient's body temperature and heat: the yang quality tends to dry things up. So dryness is yang, whereas wetness is characteristic of yin. And these basic qualities of yin and yang are summarized in Key 1. (A key may represent some text, an abbreviated slide, or a diagram. These keys allow you to follow the lecture a little bit more closely and have a clearer view of each lecture segment.)

Key 1
Nature of Yin and Yang

Yang = Sun	Yin = No Sun
Up	Down
Light	Darkness
Day	Night
Hot	Cold
Dry	Wet
Outside	Inside
Fast Reacting	Slow sustaining
Wakefulnesss	Sleep
Expansion	Consolidation

But I must remind you at this juncture that although we use the sun as the originator of this yin-yang concept, I by no means imply that the solar system is the only system within which this concept may apply. The concept may indeed be cosmic in nature. Take the example of a drop of water. If it is exposed to the sun, the water molecules will gain energy individually and then the drop will disappear because the energy from the sun has transformed the liquid state to a gaseous state, and gas has a tendency to expand. Therefore, expansion is a yang force.

On the other hand, when you lower the temperature, you will be able to transform the gas into liquid and ultimately to solid, so contraction and condensation are characteristic of yin. So if you believe the universe is expanding after the big bang, then the yang force is in fact at work. Whereas ultimately the gravitational force of all the mass within the universe will tend to collapse, then the yin force is at work. In terms of modern physics, the tendency to be disorderly is what is known as entropy which, according to this concept is a yang parameter. On the other hand, gravitational force tends to collapse everything, making it a yin force.

27

The famous equation derived from Einstein's theory of relativity $E = MC^2$ really is an elegant example of this yin-yang concept. According to this equation, mass and energy can be converted to each other according to a specific quantitative relationship. When a little mass is destroyed, it can create a great deal of energy, which is the working principle of a nuclear reactor. Applying the yin-yang principle, energy is therefore yang, and mass yin. Expansion or lightness is considered to be yang, whereas condensation or heaviness are considered yin.

Therefore, in traditional Chinese herbal medicine an herb is said to be of yang quality if it has a light fragrance, whereas if it has a heavy taste, it is considered to be a yin substance. As such, herbs may be used to correct different kinds of medical problems according to whether they are yin in nature or yang in nature.

Now that we have some preliminary understanding of the yin and yang in nature, let's take a look at the relationship between these two forces of nature, namely the nature of yin and yang. Most of you, I'm sure, are quite familiar with the yin-yang symbol or the tai-chi symbol. You may not realize that this half-black-half-white insignia is symbolic of the inner workings of yin and yang, but you have seen it, I'm sure, all over the place. And no doubt you have heard of tai-chi, the shadow boxing or qi gong type of activity that is extremely helpful for health maintenance. It is so helpful in fact, that a clinical study done several years ago showed that for patients in nursing homes, after practicing tai-chi or tai-chi chuan for a while, the incidence of falls were much reduced. The explanation given is that tai-chi increases the proprioceptive sense in these patients, and helps them to achieve better balance, therefore, they have less tendency to fall. But if you subscribe to the notion of the balance of internal qi using the yin and yang concept, then you will believe their better balance is in fact due to a state of better health. This kind of shadow boxing known as tai-chi chuan in Chinese means tai-chi fist, a form of martial arts, is based on the dynamics represented in the tai-chi symbol, as shown in Key 2.

Key 2

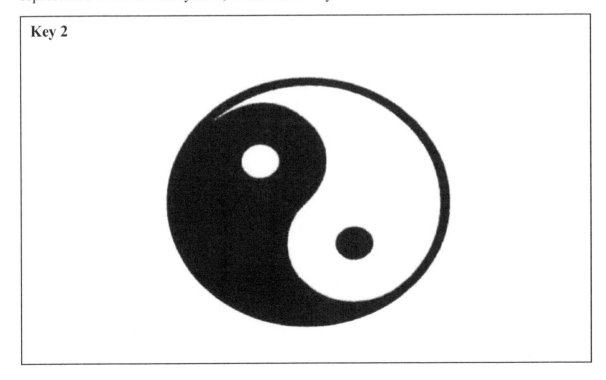

28

So what does tai-chi really mean? Tai means great, grand, numero uno or the superlative. And chi means polarity or extreme. Translated into English, yin and yang are the prime forces of nature. Again, many people have seen this insignia, but few delve deep into its meaning.

As simple as it may be, it embodies a lot of philosophical concepts. For example, the circle symbolizes completion, wholeness, harmony, fulfillment and perfection. Please now refer to Key 3. And how is this harmony achieved? It has to rely on the complementary actions of the two forces of nature, yin and yang. The white part of the circle represents the yang component, and matches exactly the darker, yin component, to form a complete circle like two pieces of a jigsaw puzzle. It implies that the yin and yang cannot work independently, and must compliment each other to form a perfect harmony.

Key 3

Yin and Yang of Nature

Nature = A varying mixture of Yin and Yang

The four seasons:	Summer	Yang
	Winter	Yin
	Spring	½ Yin ½ Yang → Yang
	Fall	½ Yin ½ Yang → Yin
Day and night:	Day	Yang
	Night	Yin

By looking at the diagram, you may come to realize a third implication. That is, whenever yang predominates, yin's influence will be reduced. Whenever yang advances, yin will recede, and vice versa -- because the insignia itself shows you that whenever the dark part of the component is larger, the light part will be smaller, and vice versa. You can also see a white dot in the widest area of the dark component, and also a black dot in the middle of the white component. What this actually means is that when yin reaches its maximal state, then yang will appear and grow. Likewise, when yang reaches its maximal state, yin will appear and grow.

According to this model, yin and yang are equal but opposite, opposite in nature, though they do not oppose each other, but rather, work with each other. So if you subscribe to the notion template of the tai-chi, men and women are different but they are equal. There is no need for the equal rights amendment, and there should really be no dispute about equal pay for equal work.

A last but certainly not least point to be raised about this insignia is that it implies the cyclical nature of yin and yang, as the advancement and recession of the two components work like clockwork in alternating waves. Take the day-night cycle, for example. When midnight comes, the yin component has reached a maximum and that is when yang begins to appear. By the time dawn comes, around 6 a.m., yin and yang are about at par. As time goes on, yang will reach a maximum at high noon, when yin begins to reappear. And as the afternoon progresses, yang will be receding more and more, while yin becomes more and more apparent, so that by the time of dusk or around 6 p.m. or so, yin and yang are about equal again, and as the evening progresses, yin will again dominate and reach its maximum at midnight. And this cycle goes on and on day after day, year after year, century after century, millennia after millennia.

On a larger time scale, the seasonal changes also follow this same pattern of alternating yin and yang. At the end of winter, when the yin force dominates, the yang force starts emerging, and this is quite evident in springtime when the weather gets warmer and the days get longer. By summertime, yang would have reached its maximum, while yin starts to re-emerge; and by autumn, a great amount of yin and a much lesser amount of yang will be present. And as time progresses towards winter, the yin force will predominate and yang will recede, and the nights get longer and the days get shorter. And after the deep of winter, yang will once again reappear, and the annual cycle goes on.

These are important concepts not only as philosophical ideas, as they actually have multiple clinical applications because these natural rhythms affect the human body and physiology extensively.

The different phases of the moon also work in a similar fashion. It goes through new moon and full moon every 28 days or so, and these cycles also affect the human physiology. Emergency room doctors and nurses often say, "Better get ready tonight; it's a full moon" because different phases of the moon do in fact affect behavior of members of the animal kingdom, of which humans are a part. It's interesting that one study has been done to show that people who are going through surgery at the time of the full moon tend to bleed more profusely, and it was even suggested that elective surgery should not be done around that time of the month. But how many surgeons actually heed this advice? I don't know. But if you believe in the teachings of traditional Chinese medicine, it might not be a bad idea to pay some attention to this principle. There have also been studies showing that the time of sunspots or solar flares somehow increase the sed rate of a group of normal subjects.

So now you may say "Well, I understand the yin and yang concept, but I still don't understand why it has anything to do with the practice of medicine."

So let's see how this particular concept maybe applied to a living world, the world of plants and animals. Let's first examine the plant kingdom. Using a tree as the example – what about the treetop? Where does it point to? It points towards the sky; therefore it is the yang part of the plant. On the other hand, roots grow towards the earth or away from the sun, therefore they are the yin part of the plant. Take a look also at the leaves. The top of a leaf where you find the green part or where it is filled with chlorophyll to sub-serve the function of photosynthesis also faces up; it should be the yang part of the leaf, whereas the supporting structures, such as the veins, should be considered the yin part of the leaf.

The yang part of plant, namely the treetop, has a tendency to grow towards the sun because it has to get all the sunlight in order to survive, whereas the roots have a tendency to grow towards the ground, because that's where the water is. Without water, it cannot survive either. So the treetop, the yang part of the tree has to be upwardly mobile, while the roots, being yin in nature, have to be downwardly mobile, using gravity, the yin force, and moving away from the sun, the yang force. In comparison, the treetop grows towards light, in the upward direction, in order to catch the sun's rays for photosynthesis to manufacture foodstuff to allow it to thrive. Clearly, the tree is a balance of yang and yin. Please refer to Key 4.

Key 4

Yin and Yang as Expressed in a Tree

<u>Yang</u>	<u>Yin</u>
Treetop	**Roots**
Top of leaf (with chlorophyll for photosynthesis)	**Bottom of leaf** (with structural support)
Tendency to grow towards the sun	**Tendency to grow away from the sun**
Away from gravity	**Towards gravity**
Away from water source	**Towards water source**
Upwardly mobile	**Downwardly mobile**

Equally applicable is the concept of yin and yang in the animal kingdom. Take a look of the human form. According to traditional Chinese medicine, the head or the upper part of the body is yang; the lower part of the body is yin. You have to remember, however, in this particular assessment, the yin and yang forces are relative, not absolute. In other words, the head is not absolutely yang, and the, say, pelvic region is not absolutely yin. So position-wise, the thorax is in a more yang position than the abdomen, and therefore the thorax is more yang than the abdomen and the abdomen is more yin than the thorax. Likewise, the back of the human body is yang and the front of the human body is yin. The upper extremities in relation to the lower extremities are relatively yang, and the lower extremities are relatively yin by comparison. At first glance, the distribution of yin and yang according to this scheme seems rather arbitrary, but in fact it is not so. Now let's convert that human form into that of a four-legged animal. If we walk on all fours, we now notice that the back of the head and the back will be the sun-exposed areas. In other words, these areas will face the sun, therefore they are the yang component of the body, whereas the abdomen, the chest, the inner thighs will be shaded from the sun, and therefore are the yin part of the body. Since we now know that we are the products of evolution from lower forms of animals whose backs faced the sun with the stomach or ventral side pointing away from the sun, therefore being the yin part of the body, yin and yang in the human body makes more sense from the standpoint of evolution. Refer to Key 5 for summary.

Key 5

Distribution of Yin and Yang in Human

Yang	Yin
Back	Front
Upper (Head)	Lower (Pelvis)
Arms	Legs
Exterior	Interior
Outside of Limb (Extensor surface)	Inside of Limb (Flexor surface)

When I first learned acupuncture, I was told that the body is a microcosm of the universe. Therefore, it contains yin and yang in much the same way as the universe. But there was a question that kept lingering in my mind – why should it be so? Why should the body be a microcosm of the universe? What's the rational basis for that? Later on, it dawned on me that this is so because it is a matter of survival.

Take a look at the lizard, which is a cold-blooded animal. Its activity is contingent upon its body being warmed up to a certain level of metabolism by the sun, so that it can be active and go seek food, so that it can find its mate and procreate, and therefore propagate the species. When the sun comes out, it must realize the sun *did* come out and take advantage of the warming effect. The back of the lizard or the dorsal surface must specialize in the absorption of sunlight, and the animal must be able to sense when the sun is coming out, so as to take advantage of the situation.

And even earlier in evolution, when most of the living creatures originated from the sea, they had to have known somehow when to become active when the environment was filled with nutrients or foodstuff, and that often has something to do with the tides, and the day and night cycle. So they had to coordinate their physiological activities with the availability of food. When food was not available or when the environment is not favorable, they just became inactive to conserve energy. By adapting their physiology to this ever-changing environment efficiently, they were able to have a competitive edge over the other animals that were less adapted to this environment.

Let's compare it to the use of energy while playing tennis. You don't know when your opponent is going serve the ball, so you stand in the middle of the court, crouching forward, holding your racket, ready to hit the ball back. Compare this to someone else playing the same kind of game who knows exactly when his opponent is going to serve. He knows that before his opponent starts serving, he will utter a couple of coughs. So he sits down on a chair and only gets ready when his opponent coughs, whether his next serve is going to be 10 seconds away or 15 minutes away. In the meantime he can be totally relaxed. But if you don't know the cue, you just keep standing there and get tired out in no time. So just being able to sense the cue, your friend is going to be a better tennis player. He will win the match much more often than you can because he was able to use his energy more efficiently.

Therefore, a living creature that is synchronized in its internal physiological rhythm according to the natural rhythms of the position of the sun, the timing of the tides, the changing of the seasons would have acquired a much greater ability to compete for survival.

Since all living things we see today are a product of this longstanding evolution that took hundreds of millions of years to reach its present state, it is unthinkable how creatures could exist today without having to synchronize their internal clock with the outside clock, which is the interplay of the forces of yin and yang, created by the cycle of light and darkness, dryness and wetness, upward and downward directions, etc..., etc..., that are dictated by the presence and absence of sunlight. That's why our body behaves according to the rhythm of nature, and that's why we are a microcosm of nature. Please refer to Key 6 for summary.

Key 6

Body = Microcosm of Universe

Reason: A Matter of Survival

And now we will look at the nature of yin and yang in biological terms. Please refer to Key 7. In the animal kingdom when there is sunlight, the animals tend to become more active, therefore activity is of yang quality, whereas resting is a yin quality. When the yin force in nature dominates, as in wintertime, animals tend to go into hibernation. When spring comes, when the yang force in nature begins to gain prominence, there will be a general awakening. According to our previous discussion, the front of the animal or the head of the animal is the yang part of the body. So what happens if more energy goes to the head? The animal has a tendency to go forward. Whereas, if the yin energy dominates, it has a tendency to retreat. In the behavior of aggression, an animal will not only charge forward but it will also raise its head, flare its nostrils, make its hair stand on end to make it look bigger and stronger. We use the expression "he or she really bristles" to describe how angry or aggressive a person has become. And of course we know full well that only insects bristle; human don't. But if you travel back in time, you'll realize our non-human ancestors may have had plenty to bristle about.

Key 7	
Yang	**Yin**
Activity	Rest
Awakening	Hibernation
Advance	Retreat
Aggression	Submission
Alertness	Sleep
Conversions of substance into energy (Metabolize molecules to produce energy)	Conversions of energy into substance (Assimilation of food stuff into body mass)

So aggression is usually associated with an upsurge of yang energy. Even in recent human history, we have noticed many examples of humans trying to imitate animals in a state of aggression or anger. The Vikings wore headgear with big horns to make their head look bigger and more yang, whereas the Chinese generals liked to put on a couple of long pheasant tails to make them look more imposing by imitating the surge of yang energy.

Submission, on the other hand, is an opposite behavior. A dog, for example, if it wants to express its submission, will just roll on the ground to lower itself, just like in ancient times, man would prostrate himself among dignitaries. On the other hand, if someone overflows with yang energy, he not only has a tendency to feel high, but may actually climb up to high places, being very outgoing, even accosting strangers, whereas a patient suffering from depression will be physically or mentally withdrawn. In extreme cases, a depressed patient may become catatonic, curling up into the fetal position, because the yin component of his physiology has now taken over.

Alertness is associated with yang because it is required for activities, whereas sleep is associated with yin. In a biological system, when an individual needs to conjure up his yang energy, he needs to have his body converting substances in the body, such as glycogen into fuel, to be used in those activities. So, glycogenolysis is a process relating to the yang functions of the body, whereas when yin physiology is required, the body will convert energy into substance. It will assimilate foodstuff and convert it into body mass, as in the intestinal absorption of nutrients and converting them into fatty deposits or protein.

Now that we have some understanding of how yin and yang behave in nature and in the human body, we are ready to define yin and yang in the physiological sense, as in Key 8. So I came up with two temporary definitions of the physiological yin and yang until someone establishes a better definition of these phenomena. The definitions are rather simple. **One**, bodily functions that subserve, adapt to, and harmonize with the yang force of nature belong to the yang domain, and **two**, bodily functions that subserve, adapt to, and harmonize with the yin force of nature belong to the yin domain. With these global definitions at hand, we can now proceed to analyze further.

Key 8

Lee's Axioms of the Physiological Yin and Yang

1. Bodily functions that subserve, adapt to and harmonize with the Yang force of nature belongs to the Yang domain.

2. Bodily functions that subserve, adapt to and harmonize with the Yin force of nature belongs to the Yin domain.

Many observations, both clinical and basic scientific that we are rather familiar with, as in Key 9, can be understood through this system of yang and yin. Let's look at some familiar physiological processes, and see if they fit into our overall scheme.

Key 9

Yin and Yang as Exemplified in Physiological Processes

<u>Yang</u>	<u>Yin</u>
Catabolism	Anabolism
Weight loss	Weight gain
Expand energy	Conserve energy
Hyperglycemia	Hypoglycemia
Hypertension	Hypotension
Sympathetic	Parasympathetic

Catabolism, the breaking down of metabolic molecules into simpler ones in the attempt to generate energy for utilization by the body, is of course a yang process, whereas anabolism, the synthesis of more complex molecules to store energy and construct body parts, is a yin process. Because this process involves the breaking down of material and the expending of energy, the body tends to experience weight loss, and therefore weight loss is yang in nature, whereas weight gain is yin in nature. This concept as we shall see, will come in handy later on, when we analyze certain medical problems, whether the patient loses weight in the process, as in hyperthyroidism or Grave's disease, when there is temporal muscle thinning, loss of body weight in association with a heightened state of metabolism, or excessive yang energy, compared to weight gain, as in Type 2 diabetes, which is yin in nature.

When an individual is full of yang energy, he is active, and must expend energy. He usually has to increase cardiac output and elevate the blood pressure to meet the metabolic need of the peripheral tissues. Likewise, the pulse rate needs to be increased in order to sustain the cardiac output. So increased blood sugar, increased blood pressure, increased pulse rate all should be considered yang in nature.

On the other hand, in the yin state, the individual organism must conserve energy. Blood glucose will decrease, and glucose will probably be converted into glycogen for storage for future use. The blood pressure will be stable or lowered, and the pulse rate will be reduced in a state of rest. So, decreased blood glucose, decreased pulse pressure, decreased blood pressure, and decreased pulse rate all can be considered yin functions of the body.

If you take a close look at the physiological parameters we have just examined, it is not difficult to see they are related to autonomic nervous functions, namely, the sympathetic and para-sympathetic. The increased activity of the sympathetic system will pour catecholamines into the bloodstream, so increased catecholamines relate to a yang excessive state. A sympathetic response is quite typical of the fight or flight response, so in addition to the increase of blood pressure, increase in pulse rate, increase in production of energy through glycogenolysis, it will also cause the bronchial muscles to relax, in order to ease the flow of air intake. It will stimulate the contraction of the pilomotor muscles, so the hair will stand on end to produce an angry look, so that other animals or individuals will sense that it might not be a good idea to fool around with this individual. Increased sympathetic tone will also increase the contractility of the heart muscles. It also increases the conduction velocity of the AV node.

All of these physiological functions can be appropriately classified as the yang excessive state.

The yin dominant state, on the other hand, will entail functions that are roughly the opposite, such as miosis, decrease in heart rate, decrease in heart muscle contractility, decrease in conduction velocity of the AV node, constriction of the bronchial tree because the dominant parasympathetic tone will allow the individual to perform functions such as rest, absorption of nutrients, and so on. For details, please refer to Key 10.

Effector Organs and the Autonomic Nervous System

	Yang (Sympathetic)	Yin (Parasympathetic)
Eye	Midriasis	Miosis
Heart	↑ heart rate ↑ A-V node conduction	↓ heart rate ↓ A-V node conduction
Blood Vessels	to skin: Constriction to skeletal muscle: Constriction to lungs: Constriction	Dilatation Dilatation Dilatation
Bronchial Muscle	relax	Contract
Stomach	↓ motility, ↓ secretion	↑ motility, ↑ secretion
Skin	Pilomotor muscles contract	—
Salivary Gland	Viscous secretion	Watery secretion
Urinary Bladder	Relax	Contract
Liver	Glycogenolysis	—

Although this concept fits very well into the sympathetic and parasympathetic autonomic nervous system functions, yin and yang cannot be equated exactly to the parasympathetic and sympathetic nervous systems. What is the reason? Because, yin and yang are far more encompassing than just the autonomic nervous system.

For instance, the entire brain can be divided into yin and yang components, whereas the sympathetic and parasympathetic are but part of this entire system. It is fair to say, however, that the sympathetic system is part of the yang system, as para-sympathetic is part of the yin system of the entire body. The relationship between the autonomic nervous system functions, such as sweating, control of the skin temperature and the pilomotive function that makes the hair stand on end will be highly relevant in the assessment of reflex sympathetic dystrophy, more recently named complex regional pain syndrome. The integration of these eastern and western medical concepts will permit a clearer understanding of the process, and therefore allow for a more custom-made treatment program, using acupuncture. By "acupuncture", I mean acupuncture modalities, also including non-needling techniques such as moxibustion. According to TCM, one may separate the general syndrome, called complex regional pain syndrome or reflex sympathetic dystrophy, into yin dominant versus yang dominant syndromes. And of course, the treatment program may be quite different. And the different approaches allow for individualization of the treatment program, to achieve a greater degree of pain relief.

It is also worthwhile noting that yang is faster responding, faster acting, and yin is slower responding and slower acting. As you might have observed earlier, the sympathetic nervous system or the yang component of the nervous system responds to outside yang stimulation, such as the heat and light of the sun, the position of the sun, or the changing of the position of the sun, therefore, the body must be able to react immediately. In contrast with yang, darkness or the absence of the sun is more or less a steady state, so the body does not have to react as quickly to this outside environment. Therefore, the bodily functions which are based on some of the functions of the parasympathetic and the sympathetic systems will be grouped under the categories of yang activities where fast action is needed, or yin activities where slow actions are more appropriate, such as the functions of food absorption and digestion. In that state, the individual organism is no longer in a yang state of fight or flight. It now has an opportunity to take it easy, digest food, and rest.

Using this concept of yin and yang, we can classify some of the bodily functions or tissues with simplicity and elegance. For example, red muscles which are slow contracting can be said to be a yin type of muscle, whereas white muscles which are fast-contracting can be considered as yang type of muscle.

You might be curious at this time as to why such a simple concept of classifying physiological phenomena and disease states into two simple large groups can somehow be beneficial in designing treatments of all types. Well, the answer is really quite simple. If you know what everybody is suffering from, whether it be a yang excessive state or a yin excessive state, what you need to do is to shift the balance towards the normal side. In other words, if a patient is too yin, then what you need to do is try to shift him or her in the yang direction. And if the symptoms are yang in nature, what you need to do is try to bring them back to a more yin state, and many symptoms will disappear. And many other categories of sub-diagnosis such as hot or cold, congestive or deficient, external or internal in accordance with TCM are mainly just an offshoot of this basic concept of yin and yang.

Now that you are apprised of the importance of yin and yang concept, let's try to explore other areas with this very useful tool. Let's try to apply our newly acquired tool to understand the nature of the hormonal system. Please turn to Key 11.

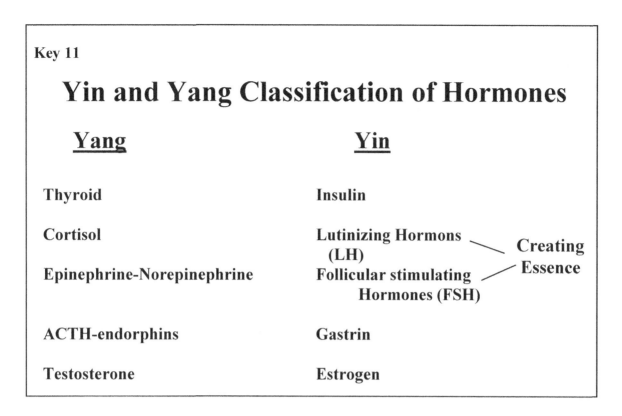

Yin and Yang Classification of Hormones

Yang	Yin
Thyroid	Insulin
Cortisol	Lutinizing Hormons (LH)
Epinephrine-Norepinephrine	Follicular stimulating Hormones (FSH)
ACTH-endorphins	Gastrin
Testosterone	Estrogen

Creating Essence

Let's take a look at the thyroid hormone. What does the thyroid hormone do? Well, it controls the metabolic rate of the body. Too much thyroid hormone causes Grave's disease. And what are the symptoms? Palpitations are associated with an increased heart rate, even atrial fibrillation. Hypermetabolism will cause the patient to lose weight, though a milder form of hyperthyroidism may be a bit more subtle. A patient may not be overtly hypertensive, palpitations may be absent, but they may show signs of hyperactivity physically and mentally. Some patients even talk faster and are more talkative than their usual selves when they develop Grave's disease in the early stages. And all these symptoms we have just mentioned are rather typical of the excessive yang state, according to TCM.

And, what about patients with hypothyroidism? They tend to have the opposite symptoms, such as lowered heart rate, decreased blood pressure, basically with all bodily functions operating at a slower pace. They even talk slower like T-H-I-S as their normal speech.

Cortisol is another example of a yang hormone. It is secreted by the cortex of the adrenal gland, which is part of the extension of the sympathetic nervous system, and many of the side effects of corticosteroids are in fact related to yang activities. When you look up the side effects of many of steroids in the PDR, you'll find many of the side effects are in fact related to excessive yang states, such as hypertension, muscle weakness, loss of muscle mass, peptic ulcer with hemorrhage, facial erythema, increased sweating, convulsions, vertigo, increased intraocular pressure, negative nitrogen balance secondary to protein catabolism, and so on. Other hormones from the adrenals, such as epinephrine and norepinephrine, part of the group called catecholamines are, in fact neural transmitters related to the sympathetic nervous system. They too increase blood pressure and pulse rate, and are secreted in a state of stress, once again related to the fight or flight response. Another hormone example will be the ACTH endorphin group, which consists of polypeptides with similar sequences. ACTH, or the adrenocorticotrophic hormone, is again stress related, and is also yang in nature according to TCM. Another example of a yang hormone is testosterone which is in fact used by gynecologists to treat women, especially peri-menopausal or post-menopausal women with decreased libido. Of course, too much testosterone either in women or men will cause excessive aggressiveness, which is as we know, very typical of the function of yang.

Well, how about some of the yin hormones? One prime example is insulin. Why should we regard insulin as a yin hormone? We can answer the question by examining the effect when insulin is deficient, as in the case of Type 1 or juvenile diabetes. Those patients will develop the symptom-complex of extreme thirst, weight loss, sometimes despite a voracious appetite, which according to definition in TCM, is yin deficiency with excessive yang, causing a syndrome known as consumptive thirst in Chinese medicine.

In non-insulin dependent diabetes mellitus, or NIDDM, the situation is slightly different, in that there is a significant degree of insulin resistance. In other words, the same amount of insulin is no longer capable of maintaining the blood sugar level optimally. As we mentioned earlier, when the body is under stress, it undergoes a fight or flight response by increasing the blood sugar level, bringing about a yang reaction, whereas insulin has a tendency to drive glucose into the muscle cells, and lower the blood sugar level. So insulin is really yin in nature.

Sperm and eggs are considered in Chinese medicine to be "Jing", the essence of the body. And Jing is yin, because it is essential in producing future generations. The hormones follicular stimulating hormone or FSH and luteinizing hormone, or LH, necessary in the production of sperm and eggs, should therefore be considered as yin hormones.

Another interesting substance is the hormone called gastrin, which is secreted by the antrum of the stomach in the presence of food. Gastrin will increase the peristalsis by stimulating the contraction of the smooth muscles of the stomach. Food digestion including the increased motor activity of the stomach is considered a yin function because it is controlled by the parasympathetic nervous system, particularly the vagus nerve, so by definition, gastrin is a yin hormone.

Estrogen, which is present in more abundance in females than in males, is considered a yin hormone, not because it is present in females, but because of its actions. Because of its yin nature, it has a tendency to cause blood clot formations, which is why in the HER study, it was shown that the use of estrogen in estrogen hormone replacement therapy can actually increase thromboembolic events. As a beneficial yin substance, it tends to protect against the ravages of osteoporosis.

While we are on the subject of estrogen, let me try to dispel some of the misconceptions about equating yin with the female gender and yang with the male gender. No doubt you have heard people say that yin is the female element and yang is the male element. Well, this concept is not quite correct, because a woman is a mixture of yin and yang, except she has more yin than yang, while a man is also a mixture of yin and yang, except he has more yang than yin. To illustrate my point, let's say a woman has 60% yin and 40% yang, while a man has 60% yang and 40% yin. Therefore, relative to a man, a woman is yin, and relative to a woman, a man is yang, and that's all.

So both a man and a woman are close to neutral, but not quite. Think of it this way: Blue and yellow are primary colors, and a mixture of the two gives rise to green. But green should not be used to describe blue. Likewise it is erroneous to call yin the female element and yang the male element. Physiologically we know for a fact that in women there is both testosterone and estrogen, except there is much more estrogen than testosterone. Whereas, in men the ratio is reversed. These different mixtures give rise to the different sexes.

By knowing the constitutional differences between the two genders, it is not difficult to realize that the concept is rather useful in many clinical situations. In our modern medical textbooks, certain medical conditions are described to be more common in women, whereas other conditions are more common in men. For instance, depression is considered to be much more frequent in women. And what is depression? Do you think it is more of a yang problem or a yin problem? If you say yin, you are quite correct. Therefore, a woman who has more yin to start with has a greater tendency to develop problems such as depression, due to an excessive amount of yin. Women are also more likely to have chronic cough secondary to the intake of ACE inhibitors. Let's pause for a moment and think about it. What is an ACE inhibitor? What are its characteristics? Is it yin or is it yang? Well, it lowers blood pressure, which is an expression of an excessive amount yang, therefore according to our understanding; it should be a yin agent. In other words, it is a pharmacological agent that produces more yin in an individual patient. And its side effects are more closely related to an excessive amount of yin, such as coughing. And women, because they have more yin to start with because they are more yin than men, are more likely to develop an excessive amount of yin. Therefore, ACE induced chronic cough is a lot more frequent in women. ACE inhibitors are also known to benefit patients with congestive heart failure. Many patients with congestive heart failure actually have circulating catecholamines, and the mortality rate in this group of patients is actually proportional to the level of circulating catecholamines. In other words, the higher the amount of circulating catecholamines, the greater the degree of mortality. And as we pointed out earlier, catecholamines are yang chemicals, related to the sympathetic nervous system. It is therefore not surprising that an ACE inhibitor, which is a yin agent which counteracts the effect of the sympathomimetic amines in congestive heart failure patients, can actually increase survival.

Another common misconception about yin and yang is the attempt to equate it with the so-called positive and negative. Now, if we use the terms "positive" and "negative" to describe quantities in mathematical terms, that is fine. For example, if you want to call the quantity above the x-axis along the y-axis positive, and anything below the x-axis along the y-axis negative, as in analytical geometry, that's fine. But other connotations of positive and negative should not be applied to yin and yang.

Furthermore, I must add here a note of caution because we talk about depression as a yin excess symptom. This is mostly true, but in some selective cases, this concept does not apply, because a congestion of yang energy as well as a congestion of yin energy can both cause depressive moods. So it is not always correct to equate positive to an elevated mood, and negative to a depressive mood, by using the terms positive and negative in this particular sense.

In this lecture series on TCM, we try to give you the big picture. That means not all the details are being filled in at once, so let's start out with a model of approximation, and as time goes on, you'll find details being filled in one-by-one, and at the end of the course, you will have a bird's-eye view of the whole system, so then you can use it with much greater ease and confidence.

So let's touch briefly upon the so-called Eight Categories of Diagnosis in TCM. They are yin and yang, hot and cold, deficient and congestive, interior and exterior. For a traditional Chinese medical doctor, whenever he or she is confronted with a particular clinical problem, the first question to ask oneself is: "Well, is it a yin condition or is it a yang condition? Is it a condition that affects the exterior or the interior of the body? Is it a problem due to congestion of qi or deficiency of qi? Or is it caused by a hot or cold syndrome?" Please now refer to Key 12.

Key 12

Eight Categories of Diagnoses According to TCM

Yin	Yang
Interior	Exterior
Cold	Hot
Deficient	Congestive

Once the nature of the disease is determined, one can proceed to design a way to correct the imbalances within this system, and the approach is really quite straightforward.

So if the body is too hot, you need to cool it down. If it is too cold, you need to warm it up. If it is too congested with energy, you need to let out the steam, disperse the energy. And if there is a deficiency of energy, then you need to replenish it or tonify it. If it has too much yang, then you need to increase the yin to balance it out. If it has too little yang, then you have to put more yang elements into the system in order to correct the imbalance. And on top of that, the disease process may involve the outside of the body or the inside of the body. Also, depending on what layers of the body are involved, you will have specific ways of trying to rebalance the whole system that we will cover later in this course.

Whether the doctor is dealing with chronic pain or acute illnesses, this approach still applies. Among these eight categories, the yin and yang concept is perhaps the most important, as shall be made clear via presentations that follow.

Among the eight categories of diagnosis, the concept of yin and yang is the single most important concept because it embodies the other subdivisions such as exterior, interior, hot, cold, congestion and deficiency (all subjects we will cover in this lesson). I say subdivisions because hot symptoms can be considered yang and cold symptoms can be considered yin. Disease processes affecting the exterior of the body are yang, and those in the interior of the body are yin.

Let us now start with the syndromes of hot and cold, according to TCM. If you open up a textbook of traditional Chinese medicine, you will find a relatively short discussion on hot and cold syndromes. These syndromes are defined by a series of physical findings and clinical observations, as you will see in Key 13. A patient suffering from a hot syndrome tends to dislike a hot environment, as the body is already producing a lot of heat. The patient may be suffering from thirst, with preference for cold drinks; there is restlessness and irritability, and constipation seems to be a common finding. The amount of urine produced is usually small, and the color tends to be dark or yellow. On the surface of the tongue, one may also frequently observe a dry yellow coating. The pulse is usually rapid and pounding in nature.

Key 13

Hot and Cold Syndromes

Hot	Cold
Fear heat (Thermophobic)	Fear cold (Thermophilic)
Emanates heat	Cold body
Thirst, prefer cold drinks	No thirst, prefer hot drinks
Restlessness, irritability	Lackadaisical
Constipation	Loose stool or diarrhea
Oliguria	Large volume of urine
Dark yellow urine	Clear urine
Dry yellow coating	White soft loose coating
Pulse rapid and bounding	Slow deep, weak pulse

On the other hand, if the patient suffers from a cold syndrome, normally he will have an aversion to cold. The body temperature maybe be low. He tends not to be thirsty, and when he drinks, he drinks hot liquid. He generally feels a lack of energy, and his stool tends to be loose or flaky; urination tends to be more frequent and of larger volume. As far as the coating is concerned, it shows a soft white coating, sometimes piling loosely on the tongue. The pulse tends to be submerged and weak. From the viewpoint of modern medicine, these symptoms seem to be rather consistent with the degree of metabolism of the body. A hot syndrome is consistent with the hypermetabolic state, whereas a cold syndrome, a hypometabolic state.

Now let's revisit all these items one by one, to see if we can make some sense out of them.

If a patient is already burning up inside, naturally he doesn't like to be in a hot environment because he cannot dissipate the internal heat. Therefore he does not like a hot environment, and we can say he is thermophobic.

On the other hand, if a patient is suffering from a cold syndrome, he cannot produce enough heat, so he will not be comfortable in a cold environment and he will prefer a warm one, so we can say he is thermophylic or heat-loving. The heat syndrome will involve excessive heat production, and the cold syndrome, a decrease in heat production.

But now you may wonder: What if somebody who is having chills and also fever does, in spite of an elevated temperature and a hot body, feel cold? What do we make of that? This is, in fact, a rather commonly encountered clinical situation. What has happened is that the patient may have been exposed to cold, and as a reaction to this cold, he developed a fever. Much like somebody living in a house, who, when a cold front came, shut all the windows and turned up the thermostat, and as a result, the house got too hot.

Now, according to the traditional Chinese medicine, when someone is exposed to cold, the exterior of his body begins to constrict or tighten up, and does not allow the pores to open, to let out the sweat along with the body heat. And at the same time, the body generates heat. So the heat gets trapped inside, and the patient gets a fever. At the same time, the exterior has been exposed to cold, and therefore he becomes very sensitive to cold and has aversion to a cold environment. So the culprit in this situation is not really the heat which is produced in response to an outside invasion of cold, but, rather the cold itself.

According to traditional Chinese medicine, the therapeutic solution is to open up the pores to disperse the heat, and the patient will be normal again. So a common prescription is to use some internal stimulation to warm up the interior of the body and simultaneously open up the exterior to make the body sweat, so the patient can recover much sooner. So the practice in modern medicine to automatically sponge down somebody when the person is suffering from high fever may or may not be appropriate, according to teachings of TCM. And one may also find similar practices were used in the times of Hippocrates, whose writings reflect that one might prefer to use the like to treat the like. In other words, a warm bath may be appropriate to treat somebody with fever, and this is rather consistent with the teachings of TCM.

Zhang Zhong Jing of Eastern Han Dynasty, one of the most famous doctors in the history of China, published his thesis called the Cold Injury Thesis to deal with the various types of acute illnesses resulting from a whole host of infectious diseases. He detailed the various appropriate ways of treating these conditions.

I must explain here that although this list of symptoms is incorporated into medical textbooks, you can only use them as a general guideline. Do not get carried away by the individual symptom, because you actually may find the same symptoms in both hot and cold conditions. For instance, you can find constipation when the patient is too hot and/or too cold, and you can also find loose stools or diarrhea in patients who suffer from syndromes of heat as well as syndromes of cold. That's why we will have the special sessions to teach you diagnosis using the pulse, using the tongue, and using other factors including the history of the patient -- to get to the correct diagnosis before you prescribe treatment. So let us now try to simplify the matter a little bit by looking at certain syndromes we know are pure hot syndromes or pure cold syndromes. Let's use heat stroke as the prototype of a hot syndrome, and hypothermia as the prototype of a cold syndrome.

When the human body is exposed to extreme environmental heat, it may decompensate in various degrees from heat exhaustion to heat stroke. And what are some of the symptoms of decompensation? Headaches and ringing in the ear are very common. Why? Because, according to TCM, yang energy is usually more abundant in the head area because the head is the most yang part of the body, right? So when more yang energy is added to the body, it will congest the yang region of the body, of which the head belongs, and cause a great deal of congestion. This congestion of energy causes a blockage of energy or qi much like traffic on July 4th weekend or Labor Day weekend on the freeways. According to TCM, whenever there is a blockage, there is pain. So when there is a blockage of too much energy trapped in the head, you've got headaches. Tinnitus in this case is caused by the same mechanism of heat rising to the head.

Another prominent symptom related to too much heat is irritability with anxiety, and it can even progress to coma. The anxiety state of irritability is often associated with a trapping of energy inside the body. Because, it has nowhere to go and wants to get out of the body but can't, the patient feels restless and irritable. And when the body is hot inside, what do you think it would do? It will try to sweat it out, get rid of the heat. But in a heat stroke environment, there is so much heat in the environment it outstrips the body's ability to sweat to disperse the heat, causing the body's temperature to go up. So a patient with heat stroke usually sweats a lot at first, and then later on, sweating may stop altogether as the body becomes more dehydrated.

Too much heat in the system can cause tetanic contractions, which are very similar in a way to febrile convulsions in children. Like a car engine that overheats, it clunks out. Therefore fatigue and syncope is quite common. Leukocytosis, which is representative of a yang excess state, is often found in patients suffering from heat stroke as well. Even the coagulation profile will show a clinical picture consistent with DIC or disseminated intravascular coagulation. When heat is extreme or Yang is extreme, it can also affect the yin, which the blood, the hematological system, belongs to. Please refer to Key 14.

Heat illnesses: heat exhaustion ➜ heat stroke

Symptoms: **headaches**
tinnitus
irritability, anxiety, can progress to coma
profuse sweating ➜ cessation of sweating
tetanic contractions
fatigue – syncope
leukocytosis
coagulation profile – DIC (disseminated
intravascular coagulation)

What about some of the treatments that we use in modern medicine to treat heatstroke, and how do these therapies compare to the theories of TCM? Our current state of knowledge in modern medicine dictates that we should cool down the heat stroke patient to approximately 102 degrees Fahrenheit using external means such as a cold bath, but it is important to stop at 102 degrees approximately. Why? Because if you try to cool the temperature down to the normal range, let's say 98.6 degrees Fahrenheit, you will have overshot, for even if you stop at that point, the body will continue to lose temperature and become hypothermic. This way you will create a new problem by solving an old problem.

Although this is not described in any scientific article, my personal opinion is that the extreme heat in the environment signals the body to try to make an effort to disperse the heat. So the entire central nervous system is geared towards getting rid of the heat and lowering the temperature. When you lower the body temperature to the normal range of 98.6 degrees Fahrenheit rapidly, the body cannot change gears fast enough, so it continues to engage in the process of lowering the body temperature, which is how you become hypothermic after an extreme heat situation. This approach is rather consistent with the admonishments from experts in the field, warning us never to use antipyretics to treat a hypothermic condition, because the temperature control center in the hypothalamus is really still normal. And the antipyretic not only does the body no good, but also increases the chance of injuring the liver. And as we shall see later, the liver is the organ often subject to the damage of excessive yang; we have to be extremely careful with that.

Now, cold illnesses are exemplified by hypothermia. Hypothermia is not an uncommon problem at all. In urban centers, older folks, alcoholics or otherwise debilitated individuals often suffer from hypothermia because of exposure. Another example is people driving around in the cold in a car, not having enough clothes on. If the car gets stuck somewhere or they have an accident, they have to walk from the car in their indoor clothing -- this can lead to hypothermia quickly. One of the hallmarks for the diagnosis of hypothermia is the lowering of the core temperature, which usually goes to 95 degrees Fahrenheit or below. Referring to Key #15, you will note that a decrease in temperature of the body can affect the function of the central nervous system, leading to impaired judgment. So victims of prolonged exposure to extreme cold, such as skiers or mountaineers, who get lost in the wilderness, might just keep on going around in circles trying to find their tent, which are only yards away. To a lesser degree, according to TCM, individuals suffering from a syndrome of the cold also suffer from some degree of impaired judgment. They will tell you that they are not feeling a sharp as they should be. Cold can also act as a pro-arrhythmic, in other words, people after exposure to extreme cold quite often develop cardiac arrhythmias, and this is often the cause of sudden death. Skiers have been known to be dug out from the avalanche, felt apparently okay and walked to the ambulance, and dropped dead. Experienced rescuers will make sure the victims stay inactive during this critical period.

According to TCM, cold impairs the flow of vital energy or qi, and when qi is deranged or impeded, many physical problems will result. Cold syndromes, even though the body temperature may not be subnormal, can also predispose the patient to cardiac arrhythmia, particularly the arrhythmia associated with a slow conduction such as heart blocks or bradycardia. In hypothermia, the respiratory drive may also be slowed or compromised. And this phenomenon can also be extrapolated to the so-called "cold syndrome without hypothermia", as the internal engine that drives the lungs to breathe just can't get up to speed. The above discussion is summarized in Key 15.

Key 15

Cold Illnesses: Hypothermia

1. ⬇ **core temperature to 90 degrees F**

2. ⬇ **temperature in CNS ➜ impaired judgement**

3. **Cold = proarrythmic**

4. ⬇ **respiratory drive**

Now that we have examined the syndromes where the body temperature goes above or drops below normal under the extreme circumstances of hypothermia and heat stroke, let us take a look at other medical conditions where the temperature appears to be close to normal, yet the condition is still considered abnormal as far as the normal regulation of temperature of the body goes.

Let us ask this very simple question: Can the body become hypermetabolic without having an elevated body temperature? The answer is "Yes, of course".

Let's say the ideal temperature of your work environment should be 70 degrees. So you set your thermostat at 70, but somebody fools around with the thermostat and sets it at 75. So your work environment gets to be quite warm and your staff will open up all the windows, maybe turn on the fan, and the temperature goes back down to 70. So the temperature has become normal again, but is your work environment normal? Not really, because the thermostat is still set at 75. In a parallel situation, your body's metabolic rate is set high, but your body's other compensatory mechanisms are able to regulate the temperature, make it drop down to the normal range. But your internal engine is turning much faster than normal, even though the body temperature remains normal.

That's why sometimes you can hear patients complain that they feel feverish, but somehow when you take the body temperature, the temperature is within normal range. When a patient tells me about this kind of symptom, I usually tell him that his idling speed is just a little bit too fast. When a patient comes into my office and complains of a cold syndrome, telling me all the symptoms which relate to a cold syndrome, it is a good idea to use a car as an example. You see, patients like examples. They often cannot understand the medical jargon that we communicate with one another, but they like simple, straightforward analogies, and you will be able to convey your message much better.

A woman patient who suffered from a cold syndrome asked me why she often felt tired, and just couldn't get up to speed. I asked her, what if you can't afford to buy gas or fuel for your car -- what do you do? And if you need to get somewhere, what would you do? She answered she would either walk or take public transportation; you still can get to where you want to go, but slower.

And I explain the body functions in much the same way. If it is cold, it is hypometabolic. It cannot get up to speed. It cannot utilize whatever fuel there is, or does not have enough fuel, and the body will function less efficiently and will try to conserve energy. And to make sure you don't spend any more energy than you need to, it makes you feel tired, so you don't just go ahead and exercise and burn up more energy. Energy is primarily used to maintain the normal body temperature.

At the cellular level, if we could ask the mitochondria to punch in with a timecard of their working hours, we would find that they would be working overtime in a hypermetabolic state, and working part-time in the hypometabolic state, or when the patient is suffering from a cold syndrome. Since we cannot go into the cells and check the functions of the mitochondria, we have to pretty much rely on the circumstantial evidence we collect through the use of various diagnostic techniques, such as pulse diagnosis, tongue diagnosis, diagnosis by history, diagnosis by laboratory findings, and so on, to assess the metabolic state of our patients.

Now let's take a look at some clinical examples of the so-called altered metabolic states, without any change in the temperature of the body. Two prime examples come to mind: Grave's disease and myxedema. The former is hypermetabolic, the latter hypometabolic.

What are some of the typical symptoms of Grave's disease? They are listed in Key-16, along with the symptoms of myxedema. In hyperthyroidism, you often find palpitations because there is increased sympathetic tone, and the heart just beats faster. And some patients suffering from Grave's disease also can develop atrial fibrillation. There is increased appetite, which is the body's attempt to meet the metabolic need because the basal metabolism has been markedly increased. There is also weight loss because the energy that's being spent exceeds the energy being absorbed. One of the common physical findings in Grave's disease is fine tremor of the hands. In fact, the tremors become much more obvious by putting a piece of paper on an outstretched hand. You can see the motions of the fingers magnified. Tremors sometimes even affect handwriting. The reason for the tremor is there is an upsurge - a yang expression of energy - in neural impulse to the hands, and they are not coordinated, therefore tremor is expressed.

Key 16

Examples in Modern Medicine of Altered Metabolic States

Graves' disease	Myxedema
Palpitation (fast pulse)	Slow pulse
↑ appetite, weight loss	Weight gain
Intolerance to heat	Intolerance to cold
Excessive sweating, skin thin, velvety, warm and moist	↓ sweating, skin cool, dry, scaly and thickened
↑ bowel movement	Constipation
Insomnia	↓ vigor
Burning and itchy eyes	Puffy around eyes
Emotion lability	Poor mentation
Dyspnea on exertion	Fatigue
Fine tremor (handwriting)	Dry hair
↓ menstrual flow	

Heat intolerance and excessive sweating are something we already discussed when we first introduced the hot syndrome. Dyspnea on exertion and exercise intolerance occur because the body is filled with energy, but the flow of energy is impeded. And that gives rise to a sensation of having to catch one's breath. There is also an increase in the number of bowel movements. As we mentioned earlier, this could be a sign of an excessive amount of heat or an excessive amount of cold. In this instance, it's due to an excessive amount of heat. The patient may also be emotionally labile: sometimes happy, sometimes sad, due to a fluctuation of moods. Menstruation can also be affected, with a reduction in the menstrual flow, which gets very scanty at times and the cycles may become erratic, sometimes even resulting in amenorrhea.

Then there is insomnia. Insomnia is a symptom of excessive yang because at night, the yin force of the body is supposed to dominate, and the yang force is supposed to be submissive. But since the body is deficient of yin, or yin deficient, it cannot control the yang, so the yang force becomes the dominant force, keeping the patient in a wakeful state. There may also be burning and itchy eyes. Again, when the yang energy or the heat surges upward towards the head, it affects the functions of the sensory organs in the head, causing burning and itching. The skin may look thin, velvety, warm and moist. Again, the warmth is due to the hypermetabolism. The moisture is from the sweating, because the body tries to get rid of the excessive heat.

As you shall see later, skin belongs to the element of metal, and when there's excessive fire, the fire will suppress the metal and that is why the skin becomes thin and velvety. When too much yang energy is converging to the head, there is rapid firing of the neurons, and when these firings are uncontrolled, seizures can occur. And that also accounts for the association with psychosis: Again, when you have overloaded neural circuits in the brain which behave like electrical circuits, all kinds of weird symptoms will occur. Just like how electrical equipment will malfunction if circuits are overloaded.

A Grave's disease patient often suffers from muscle weakness, particularly with reference to the quadriceps. I remember in the 1980's, a good friend of mine came to visit me in San Francisco from the East Coast. He complained to me that he often fell to the ground out of the blue. Basically, his knees just buckled under him, and his doctors did not know what was going on, and he asked me what I thought. I gave him a physical in terms of western medicine and traditional Chinese medicine, and noticed his pulse was bounding and rapid. His pulse rate went up to approximately 98 per minute and because of this excessive yang symptom, I thought the problem may be related to his thyroid. So I advised him to go back to the east coast and ask his doctor to order a thyroid function test. And lo and behold, he had Grave's disease. He was subsequently treated with radioactive iodine and recovered from this particular problem, although for a while, he was hypothyroid as a result. Once he called me on the phone and talked real slow. And I asked him how he felt and he said "I...am...fine." Pause. "How...are...you?" I could see his mental engine idling speed was really slow, and he acted as if even if he wanted to speed up his speech, he couldn't. And when a Grave's disease patient deteriorates, he will develop what is known as thyroid storm, in which he suffers from delirium, vomiting, restlessness; all these symptoms, according to TCM, are symptoms of extreme yang. The yang energy is very congested and it has nowhere to go, which causes the brain to be on fire, so to speak.

Myxedema patients on the other hand, suffer from intolerance of cold. The skin may be dry, thick and scaly, just the opposite of that of the Grave's disease patient. There is a decrease in vigor and a general lack of energy. Why? Because the body needs to conserve energy. It has a very inefficient engine, so to speak, so it cannot be engaging in too much physical activity. Due to the hypometabolism, the skin feels cool and because it is a yin disease, the patient tends to gain weight. The pulse rate is low because the parasympathetic tone dominates. There is often puffiness around the eyes as myxedema which although it is not a true edema, has something to do with excess water accumulated in the system. This is known as the syndrome of wetness in traditional Chinese medicine. As a matter of fact, you might find fluid accumulation in the pericardial sac, the pleural cavity and the abdominal cavity. The speech is usually slow, as we pointed out earlier. And the mental capacity is compromised, so-called mentation retardation.

And as you may recall, patients who just have experienced extreme exposure to cold also have impaired judgment. Like the hyperthyroid patient, they can also suffer from psychosis. Menses may be prolonged and excessive, with a lot of bleeding, and that again, according to TCM, is typical of a cold syndrome. They may also frequently suffer from pain in the extremities, in the back, and there is often stiffness in the joints. And as we will see later on, this is rather typical of a wetness syndrome, which is caused by coldness, in this particular instance. Hypothermia can, in fact, lead to coma as if the engine just totally stopped because it cannot get started in the cold.

It is also interesting to point out that some of these patients suffer from carotenemia. Carotene is of course, extracted from carrots and it gives rise to a thin, yellowish hue on the skin. Since this is associated with hypothyroidism, we'll say that carotenemia is more related to a yin syndrome. In other words, it's more associated with yin force of the body. And carotene has been counted as an antioxidant, and an anticancer agent. A lot of people take it as a health supplement.

Two studies had been performed to see what effect, if any, beta carotene may have on the development of cancer. Independently, the two studies separately confirmed that beta carotene, in fact, increased -- not decreased -- the incidence of lung cancer. Everybody said this substance is good for the body as an antioxidant and so on and so forth, yet now it turns out that it actually makes it more likely to develop certain cancers. So how do we reconcile these facts and beliefs? Well, the solution is really simpler than you think, because we have just mentioned that beta carotenemia is more common in hypothyroidism, indicating that it is a cold or cooling substance. So what it does is to make a cold constitution even colder. Many lung tumors are in fact yin, or cold in nature. There are the so-called hot cancers and cold cancers. So what beta carotene does in this case is to shift the body in the cold direction, making it more likely to develop cold cancers such as the lung cancers. So if these researchers were to hire me as a consultant and ask me what I think of the study before it had actually begun (something they never would do, probably), I would tell them that, based on traditional Chinese medicine theory, it is likely that the result will be just opposite of what would be predicted if based upon western modern medicine alone. And this is just one of the many examples where TCM can contribute a lot to the understanding of phenomena in modern medicine. Let's say that even if there were some law to prevent us from practicing acupuncture or traditional Chinese medicine, still, what we learned from the TCM system would not be wasted, because the same concepts can be applied very nicely to, say, the evaluation of a drug's effects, including its side-effects, the use of antibiotics to treat infectious diseases and much more.

The concept of yin and yang actually permeates everything that we do, whether it is western modern medicine or traditional Chinese medicine.

And now let's take a moment to review what we have learned so far, by comparing the syndromes where there is an actual change in body temperature, such as heat stroke and hypothermia to those of the hypermetabolic and hypometabolic diseases such as Grave's disease and myxedema, where the body temperature may not change from normal, but there are a whole host of different symptoms in association with the different syndromes, and compare the list of syndromes with the TCM assessment of whether a disease state is yin or yang, or hot or cold. We should be able to see some very interesting parallels. Since we can measure the basal metabolic rates in hyper- and hypothyroidism, and we know what kind of symptoms are associated with the two different states, hyper versus hypo, then we can easily come to the conclusion that both heatstroke and hyperthyroidism represent different places on the spectrum of yang excess, or hot condition. Myxedema and hypothermia, on the other hand, represent different points on the spectrum of yin excess or cold condition.

As a matter of fact, it may be helpful to just carry around a list of the symptoms associated with Grave's disease versus myxedema, and then start to match these symptoms with the symptoms we see in our actual practices. This way, we can form an educated opinion as to whether a patient's disease state is a yang state or a yin state, or whether it is a cold or a hot state. For instance, if a patient is already in a hot state, then you don't want to give him drugs that will make his condition worse by producing more heat in his body. As we shall see later in the course, we can really categorize various drugs, including antibiotics, infective agents, food items, psychiatric illnesses, and almost everything else into the two major categories of yin and yang, and by simply applying this very basic concept to medicine, we would be able to accomplish a great deal, even though we may not yet know the exact underlying mechanism in pathogenesis.

Now that you have grasped the basic concepts of yin and yang, and hot and cold, you may feel empowered to make all sorts of diagnoses, thinking that you cannot make a mistake. So I need to give you a big note of caution, because in real life things are not always what they seem. And you may feel that the patient is suffering from a cold condition, while in fact he may be a victim of a hot syndrome and vice versa.

A second point to keep in mind is that many conditions are not pure; in fact they may be a mixture of hot and cold, so you have to dissect out the symptoms to formulate the proper strategy to combat these disease states. If someone asks you whether the United States is a cold or hot country, then your answer would be, or should be, "That depends on where you are, and what season it is." On a given day in a year, you may find freezing temperatures in North Dakota, while in Death Valley, it could be steamingly hot. In some patients, you may find a polarized expression of hot and cold. In other words, the patient can have heat in the upper part and cold in the lower part, and he could have cold in the upper part and heat in the lower part.

In the heat-above-cold-below syndrome, you may find the patient to have facial flushing, canker sores, injected conjunctiva, red lips—all signs of yang excess. At the same time, this very same patient has frequency of urination, watery diarrhea, and cold lower extremities. So this is a pretty typical example of a heat-above-cold-below syndrome.

In a patient with cold-above-heat-below syndrome, he or she may have a pale looking tongue, a pale looking complexion; feel tired or lethargic, and intolerant to cold. But at the same time, he or she may have an inflamed bladder with a lower urinary tract infection causing burning upon urination and even urine with pus. In actual practice, the heat-above-cold-below syndrome is much more common than the cold-above-heat-below syndrome. And there is a theoretical basis for that, which we will touch upon when we come upon the theories of kidney yin and yang later on. So for the time being, we do not want to confuse you by branching out into too many variables. But there is an easy a way to remember this.

How often do you see hot-headed individuals making rash decisions, but when they really come to execute the decision, they get cold feet? So the heat-above-cold-below syndrome is rather common. You see plenty of these people around. On the other hand, how many times do you see those individuals who really can keep a cool head when their feet are put to the fire? Not many, right? So, a heat-above-cold-below syndrome is rather common, while the cold-above-heat-below syndrome is relatively infrequent. If you recall what we just learned earlier, the head, chest and the upper part of the body are yang, and the pelvis, abdomen and feet are yin in nature. So when a part of the body is yang, it has a greater tendency to develop yang excess symptoms. Therefore, the head and the upper part of the body are more likely to decompensate into a yang excess state, whereas the lower part of the body is more likely to develop symptoms due to yin excess, and that is why heat-above-cold-below syndrome is much more frequently encountered in clinical practice.

Another two syndromes related to hot and cold that should be mentioned here are the so-called cold-exterior-hot-interior versus the hot-exterior-cold-interior syndromes. In a patient suffering from cold-exterior-hot-interior syndrome, you may find that the extremities are cold while the chest and abdomen may be warm. And even though the body is cold, the patient does not like to cover up, and likes to drink a lot of fluid, especially cold fluids. And there may be other telltale signs that they are really hot inside. For example, they may have a very slippery and bounding pulse, and the tongue may look very bright red with a yellow coating, and the stool would really stink. On the other hand, a patient with hot-exterior-cold-interior syndrome may have a red flushed face. And even though the body is hot, he likes to cover up in thick blankets. And whenever he drinks fluids, he tends to stop after a couple of sips, and he prefers hot drinks rather than cold drinks.

The other telltale signs include a pale looking or wet tongue, and a pulse that is weak. He may utter in a low voice, which will tell you that the true nature of the disease is excessive cold. So when confronted with these clinical situations, it is important not to be fooled, or else you may make the wrong diagnosis, prescribe the wrong medicine and bring harm to your patients. So it is important for you to recognize the disease for what it really is, just like you need to know who you are dealing with in social interactions.

For instance, somebody appears to be extremely friendly tells you, he'll do anything for you and promise you the world. But when push comes to shove and you really need his help, he is not going to be there for you. This is a warm-outside-cold-inside individual, socially that is.

There is another type of person who looks very stern, don't say much, and is not even polite. Yet she will surprise you as to what she will be willing to do for you when you really need her help. So socially speaking, this is a cold-outside-hot-inside individual. And if you are not careful, you may mistake a friend for a foe, and a foe for a friend.

In a somewhat parallel situation, you have to recognize the disease by knowing its true nature. And the recognition of the underlying pathological mechanism of different disease states is vitally important in prescribing, say, herbal medicine. If the disease is truly hot but pretends to be cold, and you give the patient hot medicine to combat the pseudo-cold, you'll wind up making the patient worse.

So these concepts are especially important in the practice of Chinese herbal medicine. Our current course, of course, is not to teach you how to do Chinese herbal medicine, but it is important to make you understand some of the theoretical foundations of the system. But what is so nice about acupuncture, on the other hand, is that oftentimes when you fail to recognize whether the disease is hot or cold, or yin and yang in nature, you still would be able to render the treatment for your patients quite effectively. How? By puncturing the points or stimulating the meridian system which relates to the disease. Somehow you'll be able to create a balance, a normalization effect, a feat more difficult to be accomplished with the use of herbal medicine alone.

In the practice of TCM, it is not uncommon to encounter some patients who are difficult to manage, because they have very complex mixtures of the yin and yang or heat and coldness. They may have one part of the body being hot, while an other part of the body is cold, so if you warm up the body to treat the cold part, the cold part gets better, but the hot part gets worse. So you might succeed only in substituting one set of symptoms for another, if you use the one directional herbal approach. You have to be mindful at all times, not only paying attention to whether the body is yang or yin or whether it is hot or cold, but also whether there is any maldistribution of the energy. Because, only then would you be able to target these abnormal foci in the body with the proper therapy, and make a permanent correction of these pathological conditions.

One good trick to use in a modern western medical scientific approach is simply to check the basal body temperature for your patient, particularly in a chronic pain patient, for example, for patients who are not acutely ill. You have them check their own temperature in the morning upon waking, and if the temperature is below normal, which is often the case in many chronic pain patients, then you know their problem is more related to an excessive amount of cold. A really neat trick to remember.

Now let us go on to another category of diagnosis, namely congestion and deficiency. What really are the definitions of congestion and deficiency in terms of, say, energy flow? Well, for congestion, simply think of rush hour in a big city, like New York or Los Angeles. And if you are from Montana or Wyoming, don't worry, just stretch your imagination a little bit, ok? For deficiency, think of a riverbed that is about to dry out. There is very little flow, and you cannot boat on it. In either situation, whether it is the rush hour on the freeways of big cities or a riverbed drying out, transportation is a problem. In one case, movement is difficult because there is too much congestion, too much energy being trapped. In the other situation, transportation is equally difficult as there is not enough flow of anything. So there are problems in both situations, which are similar to the concepts of congestion and deficiency in TCM.

In the congestive state, the excess amount of energy may be due to simultaneous excess of yin and yang, or either one alone. Similarly, in the deficient state, there is a deficiency of either the yin or yang energy, or deficiency of both.

According to Newton's second law of motion, whenever there is an action, there is always a reaction that is equal, but opposite in direction. Ideally, the body should operate in much the same way. Let's say the pharynx of your patient is invaded by a pathogen such as streptococcus. The body sees it as an insult to the body, and immediately mobilizes all its defensive forces to combat this invader by sending in the red and white blood cells, by increasing circulation to the pharynx in an attempt to fight it off. So the throat of the patient turns red with exudate, and the tonsils maybe enlarged. And this is typical of the so-called congestive state. As a rule of thumb, the stronger the invasion, the more numerous the pathogens, the stronger the body should react. Traditional Chinese medicine describes this state of reaction as a state of congestion. And the symptoms are in fact caused by this state of congestion.

On the other hand, there are patients suffering from chronic fatigue syndrome who, besides feeling tired all the time, have a great propensity to develop sore throats. These sore throats may not be highly inflammatory, as in the case of a strep throat. The body temperature may not be elevated and there may not be a lot of exudate, and these sore throats seem to be chronic and recurrent. These findings are rather typical of the deficient type of sore throat because the patient's energy is low, and the defense mechanism is compromised. And it's fair to say that they have not too much to react with. If you apply the principles of TCM in your clinical practice to analyze some of the conditions you come across, you can come to some rather interesting conclusions.

Some common clinical western diagnoses such as rheumatoid arthritis, especially in its early phase, gout, and cluster headache are consistent with the congestive state. Take the example of gout, nicknamed the king of diseases and disease of kings, because the sufferers are often of strong personalities. Like kings, they enjoy good food and physical comfort, and because of their personality traits, they like to lead. Their constitution and genetic traits make them mentally tough, and they react very strongly to any kind of insult, including insult from a virus, a bacteria, or anything that does not agree with their constitution. They are just not to be pushed around. This same personality trait prevails in their defense mechanism, with a tendency to overreact, rather than to under react. And because of these biological and energetic characteristics, you will often find that these individuals suffer from the reactive or congestive state.

Cluster headache is another example of a congestive state. If you ask a neurologist, he probably can tell you that when patients with a cluster headache come to his office, he can spot them miles away. Just by taking a look at them in the waiting room, he'll see the typical lionid face. This full jawed individual is often accompanied by his wife, who is generally petite in body build. Now, we don't know whether this individual feels mentally and physically strong, and likes to protect, and therefore marries somebody who is a much smaller in size than he. But the facial flushing, the lacrimation, and fast coming and fast going kind of hemicrania, or pain on one side of the head, is very typical of an excess syndrome. So both constitutionally and symptomatologically, it fits the pattern of reaction, or overreaction, as well as congestion.

The angry dusk red color at the joints in gout due to the acute synovitis is rather typical of a congestive syndrome. This syndrome is also found in another joint disease, namely rheumatoid arthritis. The acute swellings, the red-hot joints that are so often found in rheumatoid arthritis are, of course, signs of inflammation and reaction, and congestion. But, when these patients become older, after maybe a couple of decades of chronic recurrent inflammation, the joints now become cold. In other words, we do not see the red hot symptoms, we don't see the same degree of swelling, and by now the joints have actually deteriorated and deformed. At this stage, we can say that the disease process is now in a deficiency state, not a congestive state anymore, because the body has reacted over and over again and has simply exhausted all its reactive power, so to speak. Now it is no longer capable of reacting to the same degree. We call this the burned out stage of rheumatoid arthritis. We can also consider it to be burned out in the TCM sense, because it is now deficient in qi.

Appendicitis is mostly congestive, according to TCM principles. In medical schools, we were taught to palpate for the Macburney's point, which is in the right lower quadrant, and the exquisite tenderness of this point is supposed to be pathoneumonic? of appendicitis. Little did we know that this Macburney's point is actually an acupuncture point closely related to the stomach meridian. And the reason it is so tender is because it is full of qi. Due to the local inflammation of the appendix, all the blood and qi have been rushed to that area, in an attempt to ward off the infection. So by pressing on that area, what you do is put in more energy to that point, when it is already filled with energy. So messing with it is actually counterproductive -- it puts in more energy into that point, making a congestive state even more congested, therefore more pain is produced as a result. But in older folks, sometimes it is not as easy to make a diagnosis of acute appendicitis because a typical picture may not be evident. This is due to the fact that older people may not have a very strong reaction, the typical acute pain may not be present, and they may not have as high a degree of leukocytosis. All this is due to their age-related deficiency of energy. So the manifestation of this pathological process in an older person is one of deficiency rather than of congestion, even though the causative agents are the same in both incidences. In the adult, or the young adult, and in the aged population, the manifestation of the symptoms is variable depending on whether the host is mounting a vigorous offensive against these invaders, or whether the response is weak, due to the lack of ability to react appropriately.

If the body follows the laws of physics, its reaction ought to be commensurate with the action; in other words, the strength of the reaction should be in direct proportion to that of the action. But more often than not, the body does not follow the law of physics, it merely follows the laws of physiology. So sometimes it reacts excessively, and other times it reacts insufficiently. When the body's defensive mechanisms overreact, they can cause all sorts of problems, probably related to many of the manifestations of what we call auto-immune diseases. And oftentimes, it's not the actual virus or the actual bacteria or the spirochete that causes the damage, but the reaction itself. This excessive reactivity can be compared to someone who has a chip on his shoulder all the time. All you do is to look at him in the wrong way at the wrong moment, and he will try to kill you. And this pattern is rather common in the congestive-types diseases. On the other hand, the individual who cannot react is like a small school boy being bullied by the big guys in his school. He will never fight back, and takes all the insults lying down, a pattern very typical of the deficiency state.

It is important to recognize whether a certain disease state is congestive or deficient, because the treatments may be different. If the illness is due to congestion, you want to relieve the congestion by letting the energy disperse, whereas if the condition is caused by a state of deficiency, then you definitely do not want to disperse the energy; you want to replenish the energy to that area. So the TCM term for the treatment of congestion is sedation; you want to do sedation in the case of congestion, whereas for deficiency, you want to tonify. Some practitioners may mistakenly believe that congestion is only associated with excessive heat, but in reality, congestion can also occur with excessive yin or excessive cold; similar to the heat-above-cold-below or cold-above-heat-below syndromes, you can also have congestion-above-deficiency-below, or deficiency-above-congestion-below syndromes. Or you can have exterior congestion versus interior congestion, or exterior deficiency versus interior deficiency.

Again, disease results when there is a maldistribution of energy, or qi. The purpose of therapy is to redistribute this maldistributed energy to make it normal once more. And as we shall see later, the system of meridians can be used to redistribute this energy to achieve healing. There is an old adage in traditional Chinese medicine which says, "Congestive states are easier to heal, while deficient states are harder to cure."

When the system is full of energy, it is easy to just let out the energy, but when the system is deficient of qi, and then it is more difficult to generate something from nothing.

A wise man once wisecracked, "Whether you are rich or poor, you're going to be unhappy," and his wiser friend countered that he would rather be rich and unhappy than to be poor and unhappy. Like money, it is a lot easier to spend the qi than to make it. That is why it is easier to sedate than to tonify.

Chapter Five – Roles Played by the Central Nervous System in Pathogenesis

When I went to medical school, I was taught many of the body's systems, including the digestive system, the pulmonary system, the musculoskeletal system, the circulatory system, the urogenital system and the nervous system, etc. What is implied in the teaching is that all systems are born equal. And never were we told that the nervous system, particularly the central nervous system, is the master of all the other systems.

In order to give the nervous system the status it deserves, let me use the *Columbo* approach. Remember the old TV series *"Columbo"* wherein Columbo, played by Peter Falk, was a poorly dressed detective in the Los Angeles police force, and in the beginning of each episode, a murder was committed and Lieutenant Columbo would then collect all the evidence to catch the murderer? Here we try to solve the medical mystery in much the same way. First we make a statement giving you the conclusion, then we go back layer-by-layer and step-by-step to show you how our conclusion is reached.

In this case, the main principle I would like to convey to you all is that the meridian system we use in TCM, or traditional Chinese medicine, is based mainly on the behavior of the central nervous system, and treatment, including that which encompasses the practice of Chinese herbal medicine, addresses the central nervous system as well. Going back once more to my medical school years, especially the first year when I took the class on histology., what aroused my interest was that nervous tissue is found in every single part of the body. In whatever tissue it may be, there is the nervous tissue. It is found in the bone, in the pleura, in the intestine, in the blood vessels including the veins! So what are they doing there? I certainly cannot feel my veins or my arterioles, so the nervous tissue must be there for a good reason.

If the nerve tissue is everywhere to sense something such as some local signals, they must be able to transmit these signals to the central nervous system. And why do they do that if they do not intend to do anything with such information? What sense is there in collecting the data? On the other hand, if the nerves are there to send signals to instruct the local tissues how to behave, then how do they know they have accomplished the mission? There must be some kind of feedback to tell the effectors that mission has been accomplished. So it appeared to me that two-way communication with the central nervous system has to be established somehow. Moreover, the sensing signal and the effecting signal must be coordinated somehow, and this process of coordination is most likely taking place at the level of the CNS. The brain therefore functions more or less like a modern day computer, because it will receive the signals from the periphery, and also send out another signal to the same area, just like there is input and output to and from the computer. And if something goes wrong in the central processing unit, then the program will not be executed properly, and a lot of problems will result. There is a bug in the system, so to speak.

But the problem of modern medicine is that it looks at every problem as a hardware problem, so every time you see the printer does not print or the keyboard does not enter the information you want, you are going to take apart the keyboard and you are going to send the printer to the repair shop. Now, how reasonable is this? I will say 'not reasonable at all' because statistically, it is much more likely to have the software go haywire than to have a problem with the hardware.

That is why, according to leading authorities of orthopedics, in 90% of patients suffering from back pain, the etiology of the back pain cannot be established, because pain is just a sensation -- a sensation expressed by a neural circuitry, and there may not be any anatomical abnormalities observable. It is therefore a software problem. So, too much emphasis on the hardware is really the problem peculiar to modern medicine. In traditional Chinese medicine, the prime problem-solving model consists of an understanding of the neural circuitry or the meridians, which behave very similarly to the program of the computer, the software. To further understand the functions of the brain, one needs to go back in history.

Early in the course of evolution, a simple multicellular organism could survive very nicely because the few cells that comprise the body of this creature can work together more or less in unison, to adapt to its environment. This was accomplished by having each cell communicate with the other cells directly through the cell-cell junction, or indirectly through diffusion of chemicals across the barrier of the other cells. This model works very well as long as the organism remains small.

But when it gets to a certain size, it is no longer feasible for one cell to communicate over a long distance with another cell. And let's say we are all cells in the body of a primordial organism, and I am located about two city blocks away from you. I don't have a cellular phone. I don't have a telephone. I don't even have a bullhorn. How am I going to communicate with you? One simple solution is for me to grow a very long ear, about two blocks long, and stretch my ear to right in front of you, so that you can talk to me at anytime. Or like Pinocchio -- I am not lying either -- to grow a long nose all the way down two blocks and set it down right next to you. This way I can detect that you have just sweated, perhaps just after finishing a tennis match, or I can smell your cologne or perfume, knowing that you are about to go to a party. And this is exactly how the axons of neurons accomplish the task of communications with other cells -- by stretching the cytoplasm and the cell membrane for a long, long distance.
So the nerve cells are really communication specialists of the body.

But a single nerve cell, a neuron, can only receive a fairly limited amount of information from either a particular area of the body or for a specific type of information, such as pressure, such as pain, such as temperature, such as position sense. And this information must be gathered and analyzed by the neurons in the central nervous system, which then have meetings, and then make a decision as to what order to give to the peripheral area. This two-way communication and central processing of information is what the central nervous system is all about.

Just ask yourself this question as a modern physician: How often do you hear patients tell you stories, symptoms, that you cannot make any sense out of from what you have been taught in medical schools? And, this despite the voluminous amount of information that you have absorbed through the years of formal schooling, post-graduate training, and actual practice of your profession? Patients just tell us what they feel. And how they feel is based on how the information is processed by their brains. And of course, many functions of the brain are poorly understood. Hence, we have very difficult time in explaining -- translating back -- to our patients about their extraordinary symptoms.

For many years we physicians have separated the patients' symptoms into two major camps, the physical camp and the psychological camp, and they are not supposed to be mixed.

Traditional Chinese medicine, however, does not make the distinction between physical and psychological; they seem to work together hand-in-hand, and we shall later on discuss these phenomena in greater detail during the face-to-face session of Phase 1.

Now let's take a closer look at how the central nervous system controls the functions in the periphery. Clinical facts and experimental data point to the inescapable conclusion that the CNS can and does control the various peripheral regions in many ways. Biofeedback experiments have proven that conscious voluntary effort, no doubt originating from the CNS, can change not only the heart rate, the galvanic skin resistance and the skin temperature and many other measurable physiological parameters. Another example is hypnosis. Put a person under hypnosis and place a warm coin that is not hot enough to cause any damage to the skin, and then give this subject the hypnotic suggestion that the coin is burning hot. Or touch the subject with a pencil, telling him that the pencil is like a red hot iron. Blisters can form as a result of these suggestions. In these instances, messages originating from the CNS markedly exaggerate the physiological response to a non-noxious stimulus.

When autopsies were performed on soldiers who died in combat, stress ulcers or the erosions of the stomach were often found. That is the effect of the CNS working on the periphery, the stomach in this case. And experimentally if you throw rats into cold water to perform the so-called water immersion test, gastric erosions can be found in these animals. These experiments prove unequivocally that physical and emotional stress can actually induce trophic changes in the organs. Various kinds of arrhythmias can also be found in patients suffering from strokes, In a scientific article published in 1978 in *Science*, it was shown that chronic electrical stimulation of hypothalamus produces early atherogenic changes in the aortas and coronary arteries of rats. These findings attest to the fact that if the central neural circuitry is deranged, it can cause dysfunctions in the peripheral organ or tissue.

Head injuries, whether from falls, auto accidents, or whatever other cause, if severe, can cause a whole host of complications relating to different organ systems. Some of these complications can be consumption coagulopathy, electrolyte imbalances, neurogenic pulmonary edema, cardiovascular hyperdynamic state, stress gastritis, etc.

There are two different kinds of muscles, the red muscles and the white muscles. The red muscles are slow contracting and the white muscles are fast contracting. But if you experimentally transpose the nerves supplying the two muscles, in other words, nerves supplying the red muscle get transplanted to supply the white muscle and vice versa, then in due time, the red muscle will assume the characteristics of the white muscle and vice versa. So the characteristics of the nerves actually control the properties of the end organ they supply.

In many debilitated patients, we often find the so-called disuse atrophy. The patients cannot move about, and their muscle mass begins to disappear. This is so because the signals transmitted by the nerve will be kept at a minimum, and the lack of nerve stimulation to the area will result in muscle mass reduction. What about bodybuilding, where the more you exercise a muscle the more it will develop, and that is the basis of bodybuilding. The more you stimulate the muscle by nervous impulse, the more it will grow in size. In a case of reflex sympathetic dystrophy, a lot of different changes can be observed as a result of simple nerve injuries due to contusion of a nerve, avulsion of a nerve, pulling and cutting of a nerve, and so on. A couple of years ago, I saw a patient who had lacerated a finger after he tried to wash a glass by putting his hand into it and by using too much pressure, he broke the glass and cut his finger. Since he had sensory loss, I referred him to a hand surgeon to have the nerve repaired. But despite the surgical reattachment of the nerve, he subsequently developed various specific trophic changes on the dorsum of his hand. There was increased pigmentation on the hand, and even the hair on the dorsum of the hand became much thicker and coarser.

As you well know, reflex sympathetic dystrophy is associated with change in the skin temperature, color and wetness of the skin, and oftentimes, even loss of bone density in the nearby joints, again attesting to the fact that the nerves really control the development of the tissue they supply. These well documented clinical phenomena are hardly sporadic or coincidental findings. The nervous system does much more than merely transmitting sensory information to the brain or effecting motor functions; it actually controls the peripheral environment, including its biomolecular environment. The extensive presence of nervous tissue in the body supports the theory that their presence is to maintain homeostasis.

Having examined these observations, a reasonable question to ask would be: Can a focus of abnormality in the CNS, such as a blockage of neural transmission in a certain part of the neural circuitry or neural pathway within the brain cause abnormalities or degenerative changes in the peripheral tissues? Can it even cause a disease like cancer? It may sound far-fetched at first glance, but is it really?

A very well known study conducted at Stanford University involved a group of women suffering from breast cancer. The experimental group of patients had frequent group sessions, and had emotional support for one another where the other group, the control group, did not. As it turned out, the experimental group lived much longer, so we can deduce from this that emotional state, which is really a pattern of neural transmissions within the brain, can affect the course of cancer, and that people who have chronic pain and chronic depression developed cancer with a higher frequency.

If brain impulses can induce trophic changes, why can they not produce degenerative changes? So if a brain focus keeps on sending to a certain part of the periphery a constant barrage of abnormal chemical signals, as in the congestion syndrome of TCM, it may induce neoplastic change. Likewise, if it sends out signals that are too weak, it might not be able to suppress abnormal changes in the peripheral tissue, as in the deficiency syndrome of TCM. In either event, the control by the CNS is defective, and the local cells may begin to misbehave.

All cells are equipped with all the available genes to allow them to differentiate. Normally only the appropriate set of genes is activated, so if there is an excessive expression of certain genes by activating them, or inadequate suppression of the malfunctioning genes, the biochemical control will be aberrant, and all sorts of funny things can happen. They may even start making hormones. They may produce substances like gastrin, anti-diarrhetic hormones as in certain lung tumors, parathyroid hormone, and so on. It appears both a deficiency and abundance of chemical messages originating from the CNS can produce equally devastating results.

We understand cancer can cause pain, but can pain cause cancer? According to traditional Chinese medicine, chronic impedance of qi can lead to the equivalents of cancer or tumor, and the very same blockage can cause pain. Translating this concept into modern medicine, the cause of pain is potentially carcinogenic under the right circumstances, and this concept may even be relevant in the understanding of breast cancers, which have a great tendency to recur, sometimes after 5 years, 8 years, or 10 years. It may recur in the same breast or in the contralateral breast. Why is that? If we think of cancer as not only just a lump in the breast, but that there is an equivalent abnormal focus within the brain itself which constantly bombards the breast with abnormal messages, then the mere surgical removal of the tumor in the breast may or may not cause this central focus in the CNS to go away, which continues to influence the peripheral tissue in the breasts. So after a certain number of years, new abnormal changes are going to occur in the cells of the breast. And we should probably revisit this issue after we have given you additional theoretical tools, as we unveil the new chapters in this course.

Now that we realize the supreme importance of the central nervous system, and recognize that anything or any events that disturb it can cause derangement in the CNS and may lead to a spectrum of symptoms and diseases, you may begin to wonder: Yes, we know about the importance of the central nervous system in the generation of diseases, but how does that have anything to do with acupuncture, which is what we are here to learn?

The answer is, acupuncture has everything to do with the central nervous system.

Various experiments have proven that the acupuncture effect can be abolished if one either cuts the nerve or blocks the nerve supplying the acupuncture point with local anesthetic. So, no nerve conduction, no acupuncture effect. The acupuncture effect can be analgesic, it can be the release of chemicals such as endorphins or endogenous morphine-like substances, or it may be the release of VIPs or vasoactive intestinal peptides from the gut, and so on and so forth. Furthermore, acupuncture is not only good for pain relief; it's good for a lot of other types of symptoms such as asthma, or the control of nausea after chemotherapy or surgery. These conditions are already established by the World Health Organization to be amenable to the treatment of acupuncture.

So far, we've talked about the abnormal focus within the brain as the equivalent of a peripheral disease process. But how can modern medicine be the beneficiary of such a concept? Well in theory, if the neurons associated with the centrally located pathological neural circuitry can be somehow manipulated or modulated to get rid of their abnormal activities, then homeostasis in the periphery can be reestablished, and the process of the disease, can be eliminated.

In reality, brain stimulation, such as surgical implantation of electrodes on the periaqueductal gray and the sensory thalamus has been used to treat intractable pain. Although clinical success has been reported by these methods, the expense, mortality and morbidity associated with this procedure really prevents it from being a commonly used method. Fortunately, the body of knowledge available now in traditional Chinese medicine has provided modern clinicians with a simple way to manipulate the circuitries within the brain without cracking open the skull. As we shall see later, the acupuncture points and the meridians, and the intricate relationships they bear to one another, put together a road map that illustrates the physiological dysfunctions within the CNS, as well as ways to manipulate them. In other words, nerve endings and receptors at easily accessible specific anatomical locations are used as switches to reprogram the dysfunctional neural circuitries in the brain. These wonderful ways of manipulating the neural circuitries to induce healing were beautifully encapsulated in the title, *Ling Shu*, one of the two ancient books of the *Nei Jing* or the Yellow Emperor's Classic of Internal Medicine, written as early as 400 BC. *Ling Shu*, by the way, means wonderful hinges or switches.

In this course, we are not only going to teach you how to treat acute and chronic pain, but also many other medical conditions as well. But let's take on this process of learning one step at a time. Let's focus our attention for the time being on the mechanism of pain. Aristotle defined pain as the passion of the soul, a very spiritual way of defining pain. The Frenchman Descartes, the inventor of analytic geometry, thought of pain as a noxious stimulus being transmitted from one part of the body to the brain itself, and he believed pain to be a signal transmitted through a cable to the brain. Descartes was, of course a genius; he was highly analytical and logical, therefore widely influential. In fact, this model has been so ingrained in the teaching of conventional western medicine that not a lot has changed since his time. So let's see how well his model works.

Based on this model, pain is transmitted along a continuous channel or cable, so taking care of chronic pain is really a simple proposition. All you have to do is cut the cable and the pain is gone. Right? So a number of operative techniques have been devised to intercept the pathway of pain, or change the response to it by destroying nervous tissues. There are two kinds of techniques: The suprathalamic procedures, such a thalamotomy, cingulotomy and lobotomy, and infrathalamic techniques, including peripheral neurectomy, cordotomy, rhizotomy, sympathectomy and medullary tractotomy.

Thalamotomy is the cutting of the thalamus. Cingulotomy is the cutting of the cingulate gyri, and lobotomy is cutting or sectioning the frontal lobe. The infrathalamic techniques, or "below the thalamus" procedures, include peripheral neurectomy, cutting the nerve directly; cordotomy, sectioning the cord; rhizotomy, cutting the nerve root; sympathectomy, cutting the nerves of the sympathetic system; and tractotomy, intercepting the nerve tract in the spinal cord.

Cingulotomy and frontal lobotomy do not actually interrupt the projection of painful impulses to the sensory cortex, nor do they change the threshold of pain. They merely alter the subjective reaction to pain. The infrathalamic procedures consisting of sectioning the cable at different levels or distances from the brain are generally marked by a low rate of success, as well as a high rate of recurrence for chronic pain. The recurrence of pain has baffled physicians for generations because obviously sectioning the nerve can be effective in pain relief, but then why does the pain recur? So the nerve must have reconnected itself by sprouting at the section site, said some brilliant anatomists. But what about phantom limb pain? Well, it is the same answer: Sprouting. The major puzzle of this cable theory is that, if it is right, it should work, and if it is wrong, it should not work. The problem is it works some of the time, but almost invariably, pain returns.

We need a new theory to account for this unexplainable phenomenon. Yes, there is a cable, but there are many sections in that cable.

As we know, from the peripheral pain receptor, the nerve impulse is transmitted to the spinal cord, where it synapses with other neurons such as interneurons, and other neurons in the spinal cord before it is transmitted upward, and may have other synapses again at the reticular formation, the thalamus, the cortex and a whole bunch of other places. The transmission of pain signals from periphery to brain is much like that of transcontinental phone calls. Let's say a call from New York to Chicago, where B answers the phone. B then calls C in Denver, Colorado, and C will call D in San Francisco, and so the message is relayed across the American continent. This is the normal way of communication. But let's say A now takes a vacation, and B takes a nap, and C, being a workaholic, takes it upon himself to keep calling D in San Francisco, so as far as D is concerned, he thinks that he is getting messages from A in New York.

In 1977, I published the first paper on the Thalamic Neuron Theory, which postulates that any members in this neural transmission pathway can become autonomous, and act independently of other neurons in this chain of communication, and that the neurons in the thalamus are more likely to become autonomous than some others. If these thalamic neurons in the central nervous system keep on sending up signals to the sensory cortex, the sensory cortex perceives the signals as coming from the periphery. As far as the brain or the sensory cortex is concerned, pain signals are coming from the peripheral tissues, and there is no way for it to distinguish whether the signal is from the periphery directly or originating from the thalamus, or the reticular formation, or the spinal cord for that matter. All it knows is that it comes from outside. So if any of these intermediate neurons -- intermediate meaning in-between the periphery and the sensory cortex -- become spontaneously hyperexcitable and keep on firing off neural signals in the afferent direction, pain will be perceived.

It also postulated that if one stimulates these neurons, they have a tendency to become normalized. In other words, their hyperexcitability can be toned down. and become normal again. However a single stimulation will not do the trick; they may respond temporarily, calm down, but get reactivated to its old state of excitement. But by repeatedly stimulating these neurons over and over again, their excitability may be permanently readjusted back down to the normal level or down regulated, so to speak. So now let us use these rather simple concepts in a real life situation, and let us temporarily leave you in suspense regarding the lack of efficacy of the neurosurgical techniques, because we will have a chance to revisit them after we have established some theoretical groundwork, before we tackle these problems once again.

One of the stumbling blocks of modern medicine is that it thinks the pain mechanism is exactly the same in acute pain as chronic pain. Modern medicine assumes that all pain must be originating from a source of noxious stimuli from the peripheral tissue, and then the pain signal travels along the pain pathway centrally.

So let's take a look at how chronic pain can be established. Generally speaking, the most common cause of chronic pain is trauma, which may occur either abruptly or insidiously. In the case of acute injury, the entire neural axis involved in the transmission of pain is activated. But occasionally, long after the original injury had healed, the pain persists even in the absence of peripheral noxious stimuli. For example, causalgia, a form of reflex sympathetic dystrophy, currently called complex regional pain syndrome, can result from high velocity missile injuries, where according to one study, 25% of the patients still complain of pain a year after the original injury.

The thalamic neuron theory explains this phenomenon by considering the source of pain to be now resident in a specific group of neurons in the thalamus, representing the painful region of the body. The barrage of neuronal discharges from the peripheral neurons at the time of the traumatic injury is of such an explosive nature that it has activated these thalamic neurons into a sustained, hyperexcitable state. Once the hyperexcitable state is attained, ordinary innocuous stimulation, such as digital pressure applied to the area in question, is now transmitted to and modified by the hyperexcitable thalamic neurons, into pain. In modern medical terminology, this is called hyperalgesia, or heightened pain. Just touching the area which normally does not cause any kind of discomfort will now be painful, such as the patient suffering from reflex sympathetic dystrophy, wherein even the wind blowing on the skin can cause excruciating pain, which according to modern terminology is allodynia; allo, as in allopathy versus homeopathy, means "different", or "other"', dynia means pain. So different or other modalities, such as tactile stimuli, which normally does not cause pain, now causes pain. In addition, the abnormal thalamic neurons can spontaneously discharge excessively, even without provocation from the periphery. So as far as the patient is concerned, he has no way of knowing that the pain originates from the thalamus. Why? Because, the previously injured part is still painful and sensitive to touch, so that the pain seems to have arisen from the former site of injury, and not anywhere in between, along this neural transmission pathway.

Frequently in trauma, the chronic pain phase does not set in until after a lag period of days or even weeks has elapsed since the acute phase, as we often see in the case with the so-called whiplash injury involving the neck and back in auto accidents. So it appears that the alteration of excitability of the thalamic neurons may be mediated by a series of cellular biochemical events initiated by the bombardment of neural impulses of the thalamic neurons from the periphery at the time of injury. The latent period may be due to slow rate-limiting steps in the chain of biochemical reactions, which eventually lead to hyperexcitability, and may be involved in changing the resting potential or permeability of the membrane of the neurons.

To extrapolate this hypothesis, any peripheral pain that is severe or prolonged enough may produce chronic pain by dislocating the sensitivity of the thalamic neurons upward. To generate more heat in this room, we can push the thermostat upward. Likewise, to increase pain, one can push the "painstat" upward. Let's compare herpes zoster and post-herpetic neuralgia, as an example. While the dorsal ganglion is definitely implicated in the pathogenesis of herpes zoster, post-herpetic neuralgia, on the other hand, may actually be sustained activation of those thalamic neurons that correspond to the involved neural segment, as a result of constant firing of painful stimuli onto them by the peripheral nerve during the acute phase.

In the case of phantom limb pain, prior to surgical amputation, severe pain in the extremity is frequently present, and may have already initiated the chronic pain process. Or during surgery, the afferent pain impulses from the amputation itself, stemming from tissue damage, cutting and so on, may stimulate the thalamic neurons intensely, thereby setting up the chronic pain cycle in the thalamic focus. Although during the procedure under general anesthesia, the sensation of pain never reaches consciousness, that doesn't mean that the pain impulses do not travel up the spinal cord to activate the central neurons into a chronic state of excitement. In the third scenario, the pain may also be intense enough to immediately postoperatively to evoke the same response from the thalamic neurons.

Another way chronic pain can be set up insidiously is through the cumulative effect of repetitious micro-trauma, as in various myofascial pain syndromes, and what is also known as repetitive strain syndrome. In these times we live in, there are so many current examples: People using the mouse for the computer, data entry personnel who repeatedly punch the keys in a high-speed operation, adding up the little traumas in the elbow from playing tennis, or overusing one's shoulder in competitive swimming (called swimmer's shoulder instead of tennis elbow), the wrist pain of butchers who constantly use wrist motions forcefully and repetitively in meat cutting operations, or the hands and wrists of dental hygienists who have to extend their arms to perform fine movements with their fingers day in and day out, or youngsters playing electronic games for too long, hurting their wrists and hands, or a train traffic controller who has to stick out his neck and look in one direction all the time, or a building contractor squeezing his head against his shoulder to hold the phone in order to do bidding on jobs -- all share one common denominator, namely, repeated action and trauma to the same neuromuscular elements, whether it be the neck, shoulders, hands, wrists, legs or the back. Incidentally, one of the major causes of back pain is repetitive strain. Legal secretaries or dentists who stand or sit in the same position for prolonged periods of time without breaks can suffer from severe, intractable back pain.

From the standpoint of our simple proposed concept, each minor ache excites the corresponding neurons in the thalamus. So, prolonged repeated stimulation has a tendency to rehabituate these neurons to a constantly hyperexcitable state, hence a state of chronic pain. Every time you put strain on a specific neuromuscular element, your brain sends a signal to that particular muscle, asking it to tense up, even if no movements are involved. One typical example is that of holding the mouse of the computer. The muscles of the forearms, the wrists, the hands, and the fingers all tense up without movement, so the brain keeps on sending out signals to keep these muscles in a sustained, contracted state. After a while, the brain will perceive this particular situation as being normal, and therefore it just sets the "contraction stat" or the "muscle tension stat" to a much higher level than normal.

This is similar to a situation where a hotel doorman opens up the door every time a guest comes in or goes out, but during a convention the traffic is so busy, and there are so many people coming in and out through the door that after a while, the doorman says to himself, "why should I be opening and closing the door when there are so many people coming in and out? Why don't I just leave the damn door open?" And so he does.

The same thing happens with these central neurons. When they are constantly activated, they learn to stay activated, and do stay hyperexcitable. So even when you stop the repetitive strain activities, these neurons will not calm down. They stay hyperexcitable, they stay activated because their "activity stat" or the "pain stat" has been reset to a much higher level. And keep in mind that once the hyperexcitable state has been stabilized, the removal of the original causative factors, namely the cessation of the particular neuromuscular activity, such as stopping playing tennis after developing a tennis elbow, will not mitigate the pain, although it may prevent further worsening of the condition.

The pain in osteoarthritis may well be derived from similar mechanisms. The major factors associated with osteoarthritis such as age, trauma and occupation, all point to chronic repetitious trauma to the involved joints. It is worth noting that the hypertrophic osseous changes at the joint usually occur at the points of maximum stress at or near the attachments of tendons. This is a matter of bone growth in response to the stress force, and usually the degree of trophic changes is proportional to the amount of stress, and not necessarily the amount of trauma. Consequently the severity of pain in osteoarthritis frequently does not parallel the degree of trophic changes in the joints. A bone spur may indeed be a red herring, merely a concurrent finding and not in itself a cause of pain, contrary to current belief. It is merely a sign of stress to the bone. Same thing is true for a bone spur at the calcaneus in the foot. If you apply pressure to a certain area, you can change the growth pattern, just as you can put on braces and straighten out teeth. The central nervous system senses the peripheral environmental change, such as pressure, and it will allow the teeth to grow a certain way, similar to if you apply pressure by pulling on a plant to make it grow in a different direction.

Therefore, it is possible to relieve osteoarthritic pain with acupuncture, which subdues the hyperexcitable thalamic focus representing the involved joints, even though the structural deformities in the joints remain exactly the same. This implies once again that the bony changes and the pain itself are both the result of underlying trauma and strain, rather than bone change itself being the root cause of the problem.

A study was conducted at Stanford Medical Center some time ago, where a number of healthy, asymptomatic middle aged man were recruited, and MRIs were performed on the spine. More than 40% of these individuals showed horrible looking changes in their discs, including protruded discs, but they were totally asymptomatic. Imagine if these individuals suddenly develops some back pain, maybe from a sprain from picking up a heavy object or whatever, then a doctor orders an MRI and sees these changes; he must think, this trauma probably caused a slipped disc, and these patients may be operated upon, perhaps unnecessarily, because these apparent lesions did not produce any symptoms prior to the injury. So we have to be cautious not to rely on imaging studies all the time.

Other painful problems unrelated to trauma but which seem spontaneous or infectious in origin, such as tic douloureux or trigeminal neuralgia, rheumatoid arthritis, myalgia in viral syndromes, etc. etc., similarly involve the thalamic neurons. This ultimate thalamic involvement in a wide variety of painful conditions may indeed be the basis for the versatility of acupuncture in treating so many painful states with markedly different etiologies. So it does not seem to matter whether they're caused by certain disease processes, whether they're caused by trauma, or whether they're caused by infections. As long as the same channels are involved, stimulating those channels through the use of acupuncture can correct the abnormalities, and lead to healing.

Now let us touch upon little bit of the mechanism of acupuncture. Let's talk about a technique used in modern medicine, which is very similar to acupuncture. In fact I have some nagging suspicions that trigger-point injection technique is really a derivative of acupuncture techniques. Dr. Janet Travell wrote a large volume on trigger point injections, but this technique was quite widely practiced in Germany, and the technique may have been derived from acupuncture in China, through the Sino-European relationship in this, and the last century.

Be it as it may, a trigger point by definition is a locus or point on the body surface which, upon stimulation, will trigger pain in an area adjacent to the locus itself, or at some distance away, and this is why it is called a trigger point. It is like the trigger of a gun, and when you pull on it, you can observe the effect of the bullet at some distance away. Trigger points are present in many chronic as well as acute painful states. For example, fibromyalgia is characterized by multiple trigger points. The triggering phenomena in trigeminal neuralgia, chronic low back syndrome, and myofascial pain syndromes, or repetitive pain syndromes are familiar ones. The injection of these points with local anesthetic or saline, or just dry needling without injection, has been proven useful in the treatment of neuromuscular pain. Although trigger points may occur at any location, some seem to occur frequently at definitive locations, with great consistency, and these points are well described in Dr. Travell's book. The comparison of the frequently occurring trigger points to the classical acupuncture points shows a remarkable coincidence, and interestingly enough, the areas of referred pain elicited by stimulating such points follow the distribution of the acupuncture meridians; we will discuss the concept of the meridians and acupuncture points later on.

Using this very simple concept emphasizing the central pain mechanism instead of the peripheral one, many puzzles in modern medicine including chronic painful conditions can be solved simultaneously, and since we are emphasizing the neurons in the thalamus as being the most autonomous, we can properly call it the "thalamic neuron theory", or TNT. According to TNT, the trigger points or acupuncture points are represented in the thalamus by specific groups of neurons. In other words, the sensory nerve fibers that supply the trigger points in the periphery feed into neural pathways, such as the peripheral nerves and the tracts in the spinal cord, that eventually project into such neuronal groups in the thalamus. So each part of the body will have an equivalent representation in the thalamus.

In dealing with pain, the pitfall of modern medicine is to treat acute pain and chronic pain more less the same, in terms of pain mechanisms. But according to our new model, acute pain and chronic pain will have a very significant and fundamental difference.

In acute pain, a noxious stimulus exists in the periphery. The group of thalamic neurons corresponding to the painful parts of the body overfires, as they are bombarded by the afferent impulses from the peripheral pain receptors. But in this situation, the thalamic neurons are passive; they are functioning as a receiver. In chronic pain, however, the thalamic neurons are independently active in a habituated state of hyperexcitability, and become the origin of pain impulses themselves. So in this case, in the case of chronic pain, they are activated, and play the active role of generating pain.

But can the patient tell you where his or her pain is coming from? Can a physician, by examining the patient, know exactly what part of the neural axis of pain transmission is involved? The answer to both questions is negative. Subjectively for the patient, whether the pain comes from the receptors at the peripheral nerve endings, whether it originates from the spinal cord, or whether it is a result of spontaneous firing of the neurons in the thalamus, the cortex is going to perceive the same thing, pain. So there is no way a patient can tell the difference.

Objectively, if a physician touches the painful area, pressing on it, pain is elicited, and the patient may suddenly withdraw or grimace, or say "ouch!" and express what is clinically known as the jump sign. If the peripheral tissue is damaged, the nerve endings become very sensitive and raw, and whenever they are touched, the pain impulse will be transmitted centrally. But let's say the peripheral nerves are functioning normally. Pressure put on that area will normally transmit a normal impulse. But when this normal impulse reaches the thalamus, it stimulates the hyperexcitable neurons representing the area in the thalamus, which then overfire and cause pain. So whether the hyperexcitability is in the periphery area or centrally in the thalamus, physical examination will not be able to tell the difference, because in both instances pain is produced by pressure objectively.

Now, one of the most basic principles in traditional Chinese acupuncture is, "let pain be the guidance for the needle". This principle was first mentioned in the chapter on *The Meridian Tendons* in the *LingShu*. What it means is that painful areas, or for that matter tender spots or trigger points, regardless of whether they are well established acupuncture loci or non-specific reactive points, should be punctured in acupuncture therapy.

The principle is simple indeed, but it ensures that whatever acupuncture stimulus is induced reaches the corresponding specific focus of the excited thalamic neurons, centrally. When these thalamic neurons are stimulated, they tend to normalize and decrease in excitability, leading to a reduction of pain. In reality, pain relief accomplished by a single treatment is often temporary, although it can be permanent too if the pain is relatively of recent origin, say.

So the second important basic acupuncture principle is to repeat the treatment at closely spaced intervals -- sometimes everyday, sometimes every other day, sometimes twice a week. We will go into the optimal frequency of acupuncture treatments later on in the course. During this treatment process, the pain relief after each additional treatment tends to be more sustained and permanent.

From these observations, the hyperexcitable neurons in the central nervous system, probably in the thalamus, seem to be capable of learning from repeated stimulations, to adjust their excitability to the normal level. This process of normalization through habituation appears to be just the reverse of the setting up of chronic pain from a series of micro-traumas, as in repetitive strain conditions such as tennis elbow, swimmer's shoulder, or electronic fingers suffered by some youngsters playing too much electronic games.

From the examples we have just cited, it is apparent that repeated noxious stimulation can lead to a readjustment of the sensitivity of the neurons centrally, or in other words, it can readjust the "pain stat" upward by repeatedly stimulating the central circuitries.

A logical question to ask then is, of course, can the reverse be also true? Can we repeatedly stimulate these same groups of neurons in a non-noxious way and encourage them to normalize in their activities or excitability, and therefore correct this chronic overactive focus by using the same mechanisms of the body? And once these activities of the neurons are normalized, maybe they will stay correct and continue to behave normally again, so pain is no longer felt.

This seems to be a perfectly logical explanation of how acupuncture works.

Chapter Six - Relationship between the CNS and Acupuncture

One of the most important discoveries of the 20th century was the work done by Ivan Pavlov on the conditional reflex, for which he received a Nobel Prize. It was now the early part of 20th century, and Pavlov did a landmark experiment by first performing stomach surgery on a dog, to enable him to collect and measure the amount of gastric juice secreted. Before the surgery was done, the dog was subjected to a series of trainings. Food was fed to the dog at the same time a bell was rung. He was then able to show that every time the dog was fed, the gastric juice secretion was increased, which is rather logical, because in anticipation of food going to stomach, the stomach has to get ready to digest the food, therefore gastric juice is secreted. But because he rang the bell at the same time he fed the dog, the dog learned to recognize that food was associated with the ringing of the bell. And after this was done repeatedly, he was able to demonstrate that the gastric juice secretion increased all the same, despite the lack of food, as long as he rang the bell. This is known as the classical conditional reflex.

In this particular experiment, what was happening?

Well, there was the sight and smell of the food, there was the sound of the bell, and this sensory input no doubt was transmitted back into central nervous system, which in turn initiated a command to the stomach to secrete juice. One can only conclude that there must be a special neural circuitry set up to effectuate all these changes in the body. And even part of the cue being received, say, the ringing of the bell without the presence of food, can trigger the same system to react in very much the same way. This phenomenon may be properly called the macroscopic behavioral expression of the CNS.

On a more microscopic scale, another famous experiment was performed by Professor Eric Kandel who is now with Columbia University College of Physicians and Surgeons, and formerly a professor at NYU, where I was a student. His experiment involved the study of the gill withdrawal reflex of a simple aquatic animal known as Aplysia. He was able to demonstrate that the gill withdrawal reflex to tactile stimulus will cease after repeated identical stimulations, implying the animal can learn and remember with its simple abdominal ganglion by simply readjusting the sensitivity of certain specific neurons in the ganglion.

Repeated stimuli can therefore adjust the sensitivities of certain neurons, and create special neural circuits, which allow the organism to adapt to a changing environment. The plasticity of the brain which allows the installation of specific patterns of neurotransmission is exactly the stuff memory is made of. And because of this particular ability to memorize, the animal is capable of taking advantage of past experience, enabling it to survive better in an ever-changing environment. So it will develop the ability to avoid harm and seek sustenance in a much more efficient way. The better an individual can survive; the better chance the species can propagate itself in the course of evolution. So what we now know as conditional reflex, memory, learning or habituation are all interrelated to the same fundamental neuromechanisms.

While the nervous system's innate ability to learn; allows the organism to quickly adapt to its environment, thereby enhancing its survival skills; this very same nervous system is also capable of learning bad habits. These bad habits can derange its central neural circuitries in such a way as to bring about permanent disabilities, as in many chronic disease states, including chronic painful states.

So we can view this nervous system as both blessed and cursed at the same time. Blessed because it possesses the evolutionary advantage to adapt and survive, and cursed because it can learn to be sick just as easily. The many overuse syndromes or myofacial pain syndromes resulting from repetitive strain are due to the fact that neurons learn to behave badly because of repeated stimuli, resulting in a general heightened state of excitability for certain neural circuits.

The paradox here is that the faults of the CNS are actually inherent in its advantages. In other words, you have to take the good with the bad. But since the advantage for survival far outweighs the problems of an occasional sickness or disease which does not severely impair the species's ability to procreate, this imperfect system has been inherited by all living creatures today.

Therefore, the old adage "Survival of the fittest" is not necessarily applicable. You don't really have to be the fittest in order to survive; just being fit is quite sufficient. The fittest individual is the one that has the central nervous system which can distinguish a good from a bad habit, and will only retain the good habit while getting rid of the bad habit.

One of the most important of aspects of the CNS is the ability to learn. Learning which includes habituation, which is a form of more mechanical learning, can be accomplished in two different ways. One is by frequent repeated stimulations, as in learning how to play a piano or tennis, by repeatedly activating the same neuromuscular elements which input information to the brain, a procedure we call practice. What happens is that you can judge the speed of the ball, so you will quickly calculate where the ball is going to fall, and then your brain will initiate a series of neural programs to move your body towards the ball and command your arm to move the tennis racket to hit the ball. So all this experience will form a database to be stored in the brain, which is retrievable on demand. So, practice really consists of setting up these automatically executable computer programs. In another example of learning, such as memorizing a poem, you've got to practice by reciting the poem over and over again. In drug addiction, there are repeated chemical stimuli to the CNS with habit-forming substances like alcohol, heroine or cocaine.

In these examples, the most essential common denominator is the word *repeat*. Learning can, of course, be accomplished another way, which is by a single powerful stimulation, which maybe overwhelming or traumatic in nature. In this case, a neural circuit can be said to have been shocked into a state of habituation.

Memory works much the same way. If you have met someone who is incredibly handsome or beautiful, you will say that this person has made an indelible impression on you, and you will never forget the face because it has made a powerful visual input into your brain. Likewise, if you pass by some very ordinary looking person on your way to work everyday, you may not remember how this person looked if you saw his or her face only once. But since you see this person every single day, you will not be able to forget the face, either. And this is similar to the mechanism of repeated stimulations.

And now let's take a look at what these habituation mechanisms have to do with causing physical problems. Hearing loss is a tremendous health hazard in modern society. The noise of traffic, the noise of jet airplanes, the noise of gardening equipment, the noise of machinery and loud music can cause insidious hearing loss. Chronic hearing loss may be viewed as the result of habituation. In order to tolerate the excessive noise chronically, the sensitivity of the central neurons serving the auditory functions may be lowered. In other words, loud noise is annoying, so neurons said to themselves, "Well there's way too much input. Let's cut down on the sensitivity". So every time there's a loud noise, the sensitivity will be down-regulated. And if this is done over and over again, the down-regulation will become permanent. Just like the hotel doorman, seeing too many people coming in and out, will just leave the door open. In this case, the "hearing-stat" will be turned down. So, the reduced sensitivity to sound results in chronic hearing loss.

The development of myopia can be hypothesized to follow a similar pattern of habituation. The chronic repetitive eye strains accompanied by sustained accommodation efforts to permit the eyes to read or look at closer objects get the visual apparatus stuck at the new setting for near vision. In other words, the eyes have been adapted to look at close-up objects, because the brain thinks what the individual needs to do is to develop close-up vision.

Another classic example of pathological habituation can be found in an experiment in which squirrel monkeys are subjected to electrical shocks preceded by flashes of light. This study was conducted by a professor at Harvard, and was published in Circulation Research in 1970. There's a lever in the cage and whenever the lever is touched, the light can be turned off and the shock will not occur. As you can see, this is a pretty stressful situation, because every time the light starts to flash, if you don't quickly turn it off, you will get a big shock. The monkeys in this experiment at first responded to this stressful task with transiently elevated blood pressure. But as the stressful situation continues, in anticipation of the shocks, the mean arterial blood pressure goes up even before these training sessions. And as this process is repeated continuously, the monkeys finally developed chronic hypertension. Again, the brain and the body thinks higher blood pressure is required to cope with this environment. And if you do it enough, it will become the norm, and chronic hypertension develops.

In other studies, a long-term high sodium diet can also cause high blood pressure. The possible mechanism of pathogenesis, according to the present principle, goes something like this: hypernatremia, or the high sodium content in the blood, produces thirst, which is followed by intake of water, which in turn expands the intravascular volume. The overcrowding inside the vascular bed causes the blood pressure to be set high. If this diet is continued for a sufficiently long period, these repeated stimuli will compel the body to learn to keep the blood pressure at a high setting, so chronic hypertension ensues.

As we mentioned earlier, habituation can also be set off by traumatic experience. In this instance, what we call pathological habituation can also occur in one fell swoop. Traumatic insults to the central nervous system, including severe noxious stimuli from the environment such as extreme cold, extreme heat, extreme humidity, abrupt change in barometric pressure, chronic worrying, surge of strong emotions such as anger, fear, sadness, assault on the body by infective agents, etc., can all wreak havoc to the CNS by setting up abnormal circuitry there. It is not uncommon that long after the initial precipitating illness has passed, a chronic state of pathology persists.

In the third stage of syphilis, when the cardiovascular system and the nervous system may be involved, the spirochete that is the primary causative agent maybe nowhere to be found. Chagas disease caused by the parasite trypansosoma cruzi, more commonly found in South America in countries like Brazil, may eventually lead to heart failure. In the chronic phase of this disease, the infective agents can no longer be found. A more commonly clinically encountered problem such as rheumatic fever, or glomerulonephritis occurs many days after an episode of strep infection from which the host has already recovered. Other studies have shown that insulin-dependent diabetes mellitus can develop after mumps or congenital rubella.

According to the current principles of our hypotheses, once the habituation has taken place, it does not have the tendency to revert to normal. As in the case of hearing loss or development of near-sightedness, myofacial pain resulting from repetitive strain may not go away on its own. So when somebody tells you that the body is ultimately smart and nature will take care of itself, don't worry, time will heal, take a bottle of aspirin and call me next year, don't believe him. Advise your patient to get acupuncture, which you should soon be able to provide, if you apply yourself and learn all the essentials.

I know that there's a famous book by Andrew Weil, *Spontaneous Healing*, right? I read the book. Dr. Weil has done a bang-up job in promoting integrative medicine and bringing into the public consciousness the importance of alternative and complementary medicine. But the title of the book is a bit misleading because the examples quoted in the book are examples not of spontaneous healing, but rather accidental healing. The patients themselves have done something right or something right has been done for them, and therefore healing occurred.

In reality, spontaneous healing does not happen too often. Just like it is a rarity to have spontaneous millionaires. Sure, you may win the lotto, you may suddenly inherit a big sum of money, but these events are few and far between. Most millionaires have to work hard to get there.

In medicine, we cannot rely on spontaneous healing; we have to work hard to get there, but this job is made a lot easier by our predecessors who have discovered some very very wonderful principles of healing a long, long time ago in a country far, far away. And these principles, ladies and gentlemen, are the principles of TCM.

Surprisingly, some of the principles of habituation we have been talking about also provide a solution to some puzzles contained in ancient authoritative medical texts. For instance, in the *Nei Jing,* or the *Yellow Emperor's Book on Internal Medicine,* one can find the following passage in the chapter known as the *Grand Thesis on the Phenomena of Yin and Yang.* "Injury by cold in winter inevitably causes febrile illnesses in the spring. Injury by heat in summer inevitably causes chilly illnesses in the fall."

Nei Jing is really the bible of traditional Chinese medicine. However, no one has yet been able to decipher the true meaning of this abstruse tenet, although, it is often used to help make diagnoses by eliciting from the patient a medical history of exposure to cold or heat. And, for all the volumes of medical texts I have read, no one has yet attempted to explain why this is the case. These are principles accepted *a priori* and as part of the very foundation of TCM. All attempts to explain such phenomena, so far, in my humble opinion, are utterly unacceptable. But when you examine these principles a little closely, you will realize they really have incorporated the same spirit as well as substance of the habituation principle we have discussed so far.

Here is the modern interpretation of this ancient tenet. When the body is subjected to excessive cold, it will raise the metabolic rate to compensate for heat loss, right? So cold injury, in this case, upregulates the "metabolism stat" or the control of heat-generating capacity of the body to a higher setting, where it now gets stuck, which, as we recall, is a form of habituation. Now comes springtime, a warmer environment, which normally would signal the CNS to set the metabolism stat at a lower point. But since the control is jarred at a higher range, the body becomes hypermetabolic in relation to the seasonal environment, and is therefore predisposed to the development of febrile illnesses. So injury by cold in winter leads to febrile illnesses in the springtime. And if you apply the same reasoning to the other principle, that is, injury by heat in the summer leads to chilly illnesses in the fall, you will follow the same line of reasoning, except in this case, the metabolism stat is set too low to meet its environmental challenge.

TCM generally takes a longer view of pathological events. So, when something bad happens, the body may not get sick right away, but it has been set up for it. It happens maybe days, weeks, or months later, and theoretically at least, it can happen years later. Because as long as the body is not under stress, whatever abnormality that is being planted will not be able to express itself. But when external stress has been applied, or when the individual is going through a period of lower energy, such as aging, such as menopause, such as the onset of concomitant illnesses, such as a major stress in life, all the old problems start to pop up. This is why it is so important to adjust the body's physiology to a balanced state at all times -- like a periodic car tune-up -- to avoid getting stressed and getting sick.

Traditional Chinese medicine and in particular acupuncture, is capable of making these adjustments before sickness, and it is therefore the best form of preventive medicine.

There is an old saying by Sun Tse, who some 2500 years ago wrote the book known as The Art of War, a book that is currently used as standard text by West Point and other military schools, quote: "In ancient times, the best generals were not famous for bravery, and their successes were not measured by the spoils of war. These were the best generals because they won without fighting a war."

As physicians, we should emulate these ancient generals in fighting the war against diseases. We should make every effort to prevent them. So when you tell your patient, "You just came to see me in a nick of time, otherwise, I couldn't have saved you," you are not being the best doctor you can be. Please don't get me wrong. All the good things in modern medicine such as immunizations, admonishing our patients to make lifestyle changes, such as exercise, stopping smoking and a sensible diet, are all very important.

Yet when you are additionally equipped with the knowledge of TCM, you will possess an even greater ability to properly advise your patients to avoid the illness-provoking effects of inappropriate physical agents such as heat, cold, wind, humidity etc.; to prevent injuries through overindulging themselves with food and sex; to stay well by having a proper outlook in life to avoid emotional traumas; to make proper dietary changes according to TCM to promote health; and by detecting early pathological changes not currently detectable by modern medical laboratory tests, while at the same time administering to them preventative treatments, such as acupuncture. You should be able to accomplish a great deal more than you would without these tools.

Now that we have covered the principles explaining why people get sick and how various kinds of disease states develop through the process we call 'learning to be sick', reasoning that if you pathologically habituate a neural circuit, dysfunctions of the body will result -- what are we going to do about it? How can we reverse this process of pathological habituation? Much of the body of knowledge of TCM is devoted to this particular task, which can be accomplished by acupuncture or acupuncture-like modalities such as moxibustion, cupping, scraping, and so on, in addition to herbal treatment and qi gong-like treatments. And since we are devoting this course to the teaching of acupuncture, of course we emphasize the use of acupuncture.

As a trained physician, is acupuncture entirely new to you? Or, so you think. In fact, as a trained physician, you have already been familiarized with the concept of acupuncture to some degree, and you have applied the principles of acupuncture, albeit partially and perhaps inadequately, using some of the techniques of mainstream western medicine.

I'm talking about trigger point injections. Local anesthetics such as 1% Lidocaine or Xylocaine have been injected to trigger points to treat chronic myofascial pain, as well as other pain syndromes. The resulting pain relief from these injections often lasts much longer than the duration of action of the local anesthetics. For instance, the duration of action of a local anesthetic such as Lidocaine without epinephrine may be half an hour or so. But the pain relief may last for many more hours or even days, or weeks. Furthermore, repeated injections may even eliminate the pain permanently.

This clinical phenomenon cannot be explained by the physiology of the peripheral nervous system alone. If the pain is coming from the peripheral nerve endings, once the nerve is blocked, neural transmission will completely cease, and there should be no longer any painful impulses. As soon as the local anesthetic has worn off, pain should be reestablished, but this is not so in this case.

So according to the principles that we have discussed, as postulated by the thalamic neuron theory, we are presupposing that the source of pain is no longer in the periphery, but rather, resides in the central nervous system, most likely at the thalamus level. And the reason it is at the thalamus level will be illustrated a little later in our discussion. But for the time being, let's say these are central neurons representing the periphery, and they are hyperactive. And stimulating these central neurons will cause them to normalize in excitability and behave normally once again. But well trained in medicine, you will immediately counter this argument by saying, "Well, by injecting the trigger point with local anesthetics, like Lidocaine, you are effectively blocking the neurotransmission. So how can you stimulate these neurons if you prevent impulses from even reaching them?"

This is, in fact, a good point, but don't forget that there is a stream of neural sensory input flowing from the trigger point to the focal hyperexcitable neurons in the brain. The constant neuronal firings of the periphery are temporarily interrupted by the local anesthetic. Paradoxically, this sudden cessation of neural input is perceived by the hyperactive central neurons as a form of stimulation. And in response to this stimulation, they normalize and the pain relief is achieved.

Some of you may remember the old TV ad by E.F. Hutton, a stock brokerage firm. The ad basically shows you a room full of people talking and suddenly everything goes into dead silence; their slogan was "When E.F. Hutton speaks, everyone listens." So if you were in a dance club or attending a rock concert where your ears were constantly bombarded with loud noise and suddenly there were absolute silence, wouldn't you be surprised? Wouldn't you be stimulated in a way? And this is exactly what happens when the afferent impulses emanating from the peripheral nerves get interrupted suddenly. As far as the central neurons go, this complete stopping of input is a form of very strong stimulation.

Once the hyperactivity is down-regulated, these neurons will take a while to return to their previous level of activities. And not infrequently in the situation of acute pain, a single treatment with trigger point injection may be sufficient to permanently readjust the sensitivity back to the normal level. Hence, you have long-term relief as a result. In a more chronic situation, however, the readjustment of the "pain stat" may only be temporary. And a series of injections repeated over days or weeks may be necessary to again normalize the hyperexcitable central neurons.

Another extremely useful technique in pain management in modern medicine is the nerve block. Nerve blocks have been used to treat acute pain of herpes zoster. For example, if the lesions are on the chest, the use of intercostal nerve blocks can not only reduce the pain, but also have the tendency of reducing the incidents of post-herpetic neuralgia, which is extremely painful and often intractable, and happens to a lot of older patients.

But the administration of nerve blocks as practiced by many physicians today, is somewhat haphazard. I am not talking about just nerve blocks in post-herpetic neuralgia, but also in many other painful conditions. Why? When the pain gets better after a nerve block is administered, both doctor and patient are satisfied until the pain recurs again, then another nerve block is administered.

So the general consensus is, nerve blocks are only for temporary pain relief. Even more unfortunate, oftentimes these blocks, which have excellent therapeutic potential, are considered diagnostic. And once the nerve block is found to be effective, then the thinking is, "Well, if it works one time, then we probably should destroy the nerve so that we can permanently take care of the painful condition." So alcohol and phenol injection is used. When it is done, pain will likely be relieved for awhile -- perhaps for weeks, perhaps for months, but more often than not, pain will recur and sometimes comes back with a vengeance.

Now compare this approach with acupuncture. Acupuncture, of course, does not involve any injection of local anesthetics, or destructive neurolytic agents; all it does is to stimulate the nerve endings or sometimes the nerve trunks.

Unlike nerve blocks, acupuncture is usually repeated in a series of treatments, because acupuncturists know full well that one single acupuncture treatment is often ineffective and inadequate in controlling pain for the long term. The reason acupuncture works well is because of the persistent repetition of the treatments, so that the hyperexcitable focus centrally will be able to respond in time. It is a way to teach or train these hyperexcitable, misbehaving central neurons to once again behave normally.

So why not apply the same principles to nerve blocks? To control chronic pain, you need more than one single nerve block; you need a series of nerve blocks. In addition to acupuncture, I also do nerve blocks. In my experience, if nerve blocks are repeated frequently enough, the beneficial effects from the treatments will be much longer lasting than sporadic nerve blocks. I do not do epidural blocks in my practice, but patients have often told me that they had a nerve block, resulting in good relief for maybe a week to 10 days, sometimes longer. And based on theoretical considerations of the thalamic neuron theory and some of my personal experience in using other peripheral nerve blocks, there is ample reason to believe that epidurals, when performed in an optimal periodic or repetitious manner, instituted before the recurrence of pain, will have a much better long-term therapeutic potential. Getting rid of chronic pain is like trying to memorize a poem. It takes time. Unless you have a photographic memory, you cannot recite a poem after reading it once, because memory, like habituation, takes time to solidify. So why expect miracles from a single nerve block? When a diagnostic block is performed and it takes away all the pain, it is a godsend. Repeat them in close succession, and you will have a much better chance of helping the patient than employing the neurodestructive techniques.

Now let us go back and revisit some of the neurodestructive techniques which have been employed to control intractable pain. Cutting the peripheral nerve, or neurectomy; sectioning the root of the nerve, or rhizotomy; surgically interrupting the nerve tract in the spinal cord, or tractotomy, have now more or less fallen by the wayside because they simply do not work very well. Yet the puzzling fact is that they do work for awhile. Patients do get relief for a period of time and these "good results" are what have trapped us into thinking that they are effective. In reality, we can resolve this enigma by comparing the neurosurgical techniques with, say, nerve blocks or trigger point injections, where local anesthetics are used to interrupt the neurotransmission, leading to a resolution of pain, albeit temporarily. The local anesthetics interrupt the nerve impulse for a duration of time, whereas these neurodestructive techniques interrupt the neurotransmission permanently. So severing the nerve is like using a very, very long-acting local anesthetic which has an infinite duration of action.

As far as the central neurons are concerned, they are simply sitting there failing to receive the impulses they expect to receive. So they will perceive the lack of stimulation as one single stimulus. Although cutting the peripheral nerve or tract is a very, very strong stimulus, they may respond by temporarily adjusting their pain stat downward to a normal level, and therefore the patient experiences relief of pain.

But as time goes on, the down-regulated pain stat is going to bounce back up to its previously abnormal level because a single strong stimulation is really not quite sufficient to permanently adjust its activity. So the recurrence of the pain is more of a rule than an exception. So if you don't cut the nerve, you actually preserve a pathway through which you can modulate these abnormal mechanisms by doing multiple nerve blocks, multiple trigger point injections at the same site on a recurrent basis, so that you can accumulate all the effects of the individual stimulations, with the hope of permanently correcting the pathological focus.

The neural destructive techniques are like a single nerve block, a single powerful stimulation that may or may not succeed. And if it does not succeed, then a pathway useful for neural modulation will be lost permanently. By the same token, the preliminary test blocking of a branch of a trigeminal nerve with anesthetic agents before neurectomy in the treatment of tic douloureaux, may indeed be a far superior therapeutic modality than the neurodestructive technique itself, if the nerve block is repeated over and over again. Aside from the inevitable morbidity, most forms of neurodestruction are unsatisfactory in accomplishing long lasting relief, because they do not provide the repetitious stimuli necessary to habituate or reset the neuronal pain stat.

Back operations are much more common than neurosurgery in the treatment of pain, and a very significant number of patients do not respond well to back surgeries such as laminectomy; the same concept we have been discussing can also be extrapolated theoretically to these conditions. We kept on doing these surgeries because a good number patients do respond well to these operations, and this is what led us to believe, perhaps mistakenly, that we must have been doing something absolutely right. If you look closely, the therapeutic effect of surgical operation is very similar to that of acupuncture, although surgeons probably will disagree strongly with me -- because the cutting, removal or manipulation of tissues create very strong neural input in the central nervous system, in a corresponding area of the brain that represents the peripheral part that has been operated upon, and this very strong stimulation bears close resemblance to those of the neurosurgical techniques that we have been talking about. Such strong stimulation can equally effectuate changes in the centrally located pathological focus, causing its abnormal neuronal activities to normalize.

The destruction of tissue can actually arouse a healing process within the body itself. This is evidenced by the technique known as direct moxibustion, where the dry leaves of an herbal plant called artemisia vulgaris, rolled into a fine wool is sometimes burned directly on the skin, creating a scar; this method serves in the treatment of certain intractable medical conditions including chronic recalcitrant pain.

In modern medicine, back operations do not always work, and the patient may experience recurrent pain. These are then known as the failed back syndromes. And oftentimes, these patients have again undergone surgery, which again gave them a temporary reprieve followed again by return of symptoms. In retrospect perhaps, these patients should have received neural modulation therapy, a term I have used for more than 25 years, which includes acupuncture and acupuncture-related therapeutics and which could have done more good for these patients.

Let me give you a real life example of a patient who happens to be a physician as well. Several years ago, this patient developed right-sided neck pain, and an MRI showed that she had a protruded disc at the lower cervical level. What is interesting is that her pain was on the right side, but the disc was protruded to the left, so the objective findings seemed to be inconsistent to her symptomatology. Nevertheless, surgery was proposed and she consented, that's before she came to see me. A few years after the surgery she still had a considerable amount of pain, although the pain was not as severe as before she had the surgery. Now what you make of that?

The pieces of this jigsaw puzzle don't seem to fit. so when she came to me for acupuncture treatment to relieve her pain and ask me how I interpreted all these findings, I gave her the following explanations after I had performed a complete history and physical, and noted there was considerable amount of spasm in the paraspinal muscles on the right side in the cervical as well as the thoracic regions.

The pain originated from the muscle group on the right-hand side. A chronic contraction of these muscles has the tendency of squeezing out the disc towards the left side. Much like if you hold a Big Mac, a McDonald's hamburger, with one hand long enough, it has the tendency to squeeze the beef patty towards the other side. The hamburger patty in this case is like the disc, and the buns on top and below the patty are similar to the vertebral bodies on top of and below the disc. When a chronic force has been exerted on the nucleus propulsus, it can dislocate, just like when you put braces on teeth, they will grow in a certain direction, a key principle in orthodontics. This should also happen if the different muscles along the spine contract with different forces; these imbalances may have accounted for the awful pictures seen on MRI of a whole bunch of normal, asymptomatic middle-aged men in the Stanford study.

So the disc herniated to the left side may in fact has been the result, rather than the cause, of her pain. The cause of the pain was on the right side, causing the muscle spasm, or maybe a result of the muscle spasm. But in any event, it was a right-sided problem, but the disc operation on the left side did help her. This is so because it is sort of like a very good acupuncture treatment right next to the midline of the spine, which can affect an area surrounding this particular focus and have the ability to normalize some of the abnormally functioning neurons in the central nervous system that represent the muscles on the right side, inducing partial pain relief. With a short course of acupuncture treatment along with Chinese herbal treatment, she did get quite a bit of relief from this rather incapacitating condition, lending support to the assessment we have just described.

Now it is perhaps a good time to revisit some of the issues relating to breast cancer. As we recall, breast cancer has a strong tendency to recur, and the five year survival is no guarantee that it won't come back ten years later, say. Why is that so?

The recurrence is not necessarily caused by some tumor cells being left in the area due to incomplete surgical removal of the tumor, because according to the thalamic neuron theory concept, there is an equivalent abnormal focus in the brain itself, which ultimately controls the trophic changes in the peripheral tissues such as the breast.

If this abnormal focus keeps on sending off messages to the tissue causing the abnormal gene to express itself and finally trigger the cells to transform into a tumor, then there is breast cancer. But this process may have taken a long time to develop. So when the cancer is removed from the breast surgically with concomitant radiation therapy, that area of the breast has received a very strong stimulation. This stimulation is translated into a normalizing impulse that got fed into the abnormal focus into the brain, causing it to normalize. And if successful, then the problem is gone forever. But let's say this normalization process is only partial -- then this abnormal focus will behave for a while, only to revert to its old self after some time, maybe a few years. Or it may not have changed at all. In either event, it will resume bombarding the periphery with abnormal messages immediately or later on, and the cumulative effect of these abnormal efferent controls eventually turn some of the breast cells into cancer cells once more. And since these centrally originating abnormal impulses may hit the left breast or the right breast, the recurrence may be seen in the same breast or on the contralateral breast.

This concept also accounts for the influence of the emotional state on the course of disease, including cancer, because emotion is nothing more than a specific pattern of neural activities. A good mental attitude is certainly helpful for healing. Based on the theoretical considerations of the TNT, I actually proposed in a paper that I wrote in 1994 a brand new approach to the treatment of cancers, especially metastatic cancer. Applying what we have learned so far, you can categorize cancer into different groups, the congestive type of cancers versus the deficient type of cancers, versus hot cancers or cold cancers. Perhaps the congestive type of cancers will be more amenable to surgical intervention, not in terms of removal of cancer tissues as you might expect, but in terms of stimulating the abnormal areas where cancer is found.

So here is the 6 million dollar question: If repetitious stimulation is the key in the treatment of chronic diseases, might cancer that has spread be treated the same way?

According the thalamic neuron theory, a pathological neuronal focus must simultaneously exist in the brain, as the cancer cells in the periphery. The therapeutic objective will be to convert these neurons of abnormal activities back to normal, in order that peripheral homeostasis be re-established. As we said, surgery which involves cutting and removal of tissues is in and of itself a strong stimulation. A cancer is considered inoperable if it has spread diffusely and all of the cancer cells cannot be surgically removed. However, the complete removal of all the cancer cells at once may not be necessary in order for the patient to benefit from the procedure, from the viewpoint of TNT. As each discrete mass of tumor is removed, a strong stimulation is delivered to the abnormal focus within the brain to initiate a normalizing trend, but if permanent benefit is to be obtained, surgery must be repeated, with additional cancerous tissues removed each time, to dehabituate and normalize the abnormal focus on a long-term basis. Concurrent with the series of operations, the body should be fortified by other adjunctive therapies such as Chinese herbal medicine, acupuncture and so on. It may not be necessary to remove all the cancerous tissues at once or remove them completely because practically, this may not be feasible. The prediction is the patient still may benefit, and survival may be significantly prolonged.

Within this context, I believe a final topic should be a theoretical assessment of many of the new drugs to be developed for different kinds of medical conditions. Unless we realize the controlling mechanism of the CNS in many disease processes, many of these drug regimens will fail. Many modern drug therapies take care of only the peripheral manifestation of the symptoms by either suppressing the symptoms or neutralizing them, but without actually counteracting them at the origin. It's like the thermostat in this room is bumped up to 85 degrees: It gets very hot so you open up the window, turn on the fan and does get rid of the heat, and sure, the temperature will be lowered. But you have not really taken care of the problem; the thermostat is still set at 85. As long as you turn off the fan and shut the windows, the temperature will go up once more.

In a disease like Type II diabetes, sulfonylurea is used to force the islet cells in the pancreas to release insulin, without caring for why it is not released in the first place. What signals have been messed up in the brain? And drugs like Metformin help to sensitize insulin without correcting the underlying reason that insulin resistance developed in the first place.

So, good control of the blood sugar, which is one of the many manifestations of diabetes may not be able to prevent all the complications of this disease. Some of the endocrine diseases, noticeably diabetes mellitus and Grave's disease, can be viewed as diseases of the CNS with peripheral manifestations, each involving one primary target endocrine organ, namely the pancreas and the thyroid respectively.

The control of symptoms cannot be equated to the ability to prevent certain complications, such as retinopathy, despite reasonably good control of blood sugar levels. Diabetes can be thought of as a CNS disease affecting multiple organ systems, even though many important symptoms are associated with the lack of insulin from the pancreas.

Likewise, Grave's disease can be treated by destroying part of the thyroid gland with radioactive iodine, but sometimes exophthalmus or the protrusion of the eyes, another prominent symptom of hyperthyroidism, continues to progress despite a normal functioning thyroid gland following treatment. In both diseases, the endocrine dysfunction is only part of, albeit an important part of, the total clinical picture, as the replacement of insulin or the destruction of the thyroid gland does not necessarily normalize the pathological neural circuitries within the CNS, and the diseases continue to progress, and affect other target tissues and organs.

The onset of insulin-dependent diabetes in children is not uncommonly preceded by an episode of an infection such as mumps, and the onset of Grave's disease is often preceded by major emotional crisis or traumatic experience. In both cases, the CNS is involved according to the present theory, and the controlling neural circuitries are shocked into disarray, perpetuating pathological processes.

In the pharmaceutical arena, many new drugs have been developed to treat infections, because bacterial resistance to antibiotics is a fast emerging and serious problem all over the world. It is a virtual race between the bacteria's mutating into ever more resistant strains, and our newest antibiotics. We may soon run out of effective regimens to treat very serious illnesses. Among the prominent players are the strep pneumoniae, MRSA, (Methicillin-resistant Staphylococcus aureus), and VRE, (Vancomycin-Resistant Enterococci).

But in any infectious disease, there are two components to the equation, namely the infective agent and the host. All the efforts have been concentrated so far on killing off the invading organism, the bacteria, the bad guys. But in the modern western therapeutic armamentarium, few agents are available to strengthen the host's defense. The pharmaceutical companies have turned out anti-HIV drugs by the dozen, in an attempt to eliminate HIV, and have wound up having to deal with many of the serious side effects, without a clear-cut victory over this deadly enemy of the human race.

So what are we to do? Some of the potential answers lie within the realm of TCM; where agents abound and are available to tonify the human body, to increase the immune response. Already there are some preliminary test projects that show promise in modifying the course of the disease, but many potential effective treatments have really not been tried.

Similarly, traditional Chinese medicines has been used successfully to treat tuberculosis, and when Chinese therapeutic formulae are combined with western drug therapy, a better outcome may be at hand, especially when dealing with resistant strains of the tuberculosis bacilli.

President Kennedy in his inaugural speech said, "Ask not what your country can do for you; ask what you can do for your country." And in much the same spirit, I will say to you, "Ask not what modern medicine can do for traditional Chinese medicine; ask what traditional Chinese medicine can do for modern medicine".

Sure, it may be important, but we should not let ourselves get bogged down by trying to exclusively use western methodology to prove or explain how acupuncture works on each particular disease entity, but rather we should utilize the teachings of traditional Chinese medicine as tools and insights to develop new ways of thinking, and ask new questions, and develop new concepts, to make modern medicine much more effective. And this is why we have emphasized the presentation of the above concepts.

Chapter Seven – The Concept of Kidney Deficiency

You might think the system of Chinese medicine is a complete, integrative system of knowledge where everybody agrees with everybody else, and that there is a consensus about the approach to the treatment of diseases, and there is no dispute about the basic concepts.

Well, you're wrong, I'm sorry to say. Fortunately for the individual patient, these differences in opinion about the overall concept do not radically alter the therapeutic approach for that particular patient.

We have already spent some time reviewing the yin and yang concepts in terms of not only traditional Chinese medicine, but in terms of the biological world and nature itself. Since we already have some global understanding of how yin and yang work, we are ready to tackle a more specific study of the finer implications of this concept in providing treatments such as acupuncture. Let's now take a closer look at the focal point of a historical dispute.

Zhu Danxi, a famous physician who lived from 1282 to 1358 AD, maintained that the yang of the body tends to be excessive, and the yin tends to be deficient, and he was famous for his methodology of using cooling therapeutic agents in the Chinese medicine armamentarium to treat a variety of hot conditions. Zhang Jing Yueh who lived about 300 years after Zhu Danxi during the Ming Dynasty, strongly disagreed with his assessment about the body's tendency to have yang excess and yin deficiency. According to him, yang is never excessive and yin is frequently deficient.

Now, both of these doctors are historically famous. They had a lot to contribute to the understanding of using therapeutic agents. They both wrote voluminous amounts of literatures on Chinese medicine. So who is right? So they have us scratching our heads.

But don't worry. Before the day is over, you will have a clear understanding of what they're talking about, and will gain a proper understanding of this very important TCM concept in terms of modern medicine, better than many TCM practitioners in the field, because the solution to this puzzle is both logical and supported by ample experimental evidence.

Despite the popularity of alternative medicine or complementary medicine or integrative medicine, the medical community of the western world still experiences great difficulty in wholeheartedly endorsing the use of traditional Chinese medical modalities, including acupuncture, moxibustion, herbal and other therapeutic agents, primarily due to the lack of reasonable scientific interpretations of many of the traditional Chinese medical concepts within the context of modern medicine. Therapeutic principles of Chinese medicine appear largely abstract and untenable to modern physicians; as philosophical explanations are far from convincing, they just don't get it at the gut level.

In contrast to these inscrutable Chinese medicine principles, the efficacy of various therapeutic modalities of TCM, particularly acupuncture, remains an objective fact. It is extremely important, therefore, to translate these abstruse Chinese medical notions into concrete modern scientific terms.

The concept of kidney deficiency is among the most important notions in traditional Chinese medicine, and has received in recent years a good deal of scientific attention in China. There's a lot of investigative work that has already been done to correlate the syndromes of kidney deficiency in the traditional Chinese medical sense with objective physical and biochemical findings. The experimental data and clinical experience with kidney deficiency syndromes have been nicely summarized in the monogram called *Combined Chinese and Modern Medical Therapy in the Treatment of Kidney Deficiency Syndromes* by Tian Hua, et al., of the First Medical College of Shanghai in China. To summarize the most valuable information concerning kidney deficiency syndromes obtained so far are the following points: (Please refer to Key K-1, Key K-2.)

Key K-1,
Key K-2

Symptoms and Signs of Kidney Qi Deficiency

Kidney Yin Deficiency Key K-1	**Kidney Yang Deficiency** Key K-2
Symptoms: Breathlessness	Aversion to Cold environment
Irritability	Edema
Feverishness	Diarrhea
Dry mouth	Increase volume of urination
Dizziness	Increase frequency of urination
Visual disturbance	Easy fatigability
Tinnitus	Shortness of breath
Night sweat	Sexual impotence
Insomnia	Lowback ache
Constipation	Weakness in extremities
Dysuria	Nocturnal Emission
❖　　　　❖	❖　　　　❖
Signs: Bright red tongue	Wet bulky tongue, pale tongue
Patchy, cracked coating	Slow deep weak
Fast, small pulse	(submerged) pulse

87

Point #1 – The kidney system, according to traditional Chinese medicine, involves a series of physiological phenomena and processes which are functionally but not necessarily anatomically related to the kidney organ, or more precisely, the urogenital system.

The "kidney functions" can be classified into a yin and a yang component. Symptoms and signs of kidney yin deficiency include, as outlined in Key K-1, breathlessness, irritability, feverishness, dry mouth, dizziness, visual disturbance, tinnitus, night sweats, insomnia, constipation, dysuria or burning urination, nocturnal emission, and a bright red tongue with a patchy or cracked coating, along with a fast and small pulse.

On the other side, the symptoms and signs of kidney yang deficiency include a strong dislike of a cold environment, edema or swelling with fluid accumulation, diarrhea, increased volume and frequency of urination, easy fatiguability, shortness of breath, sexual impotence, low back ache, a wet looking tongue, and a slow-deep pulse. Additionally, there is achiness associated with a tired sensation in the lower back, weakness in the extremities, hair shredding, loose teeth and a weak chueh pulse (see Key K-2).

Chueh pulse is the proximal pulse at one of the three positions of the radial artery near the wrist.

These symptoms and physical findings can occur in both the yin deficient and the yang deficient states. Take a look at these symptoms and you will find that they correlate more or less with the ones that we mentioned earlier during the talk on yin and yang symptoms. The reason for this parallel comparison is due to the fact that the kidney is the leader of all other systems; similar to the nervous system being the commander of all other physiological systems,, the kidney system and the brain are considered to be one extended system in TCM. We also mentioned earlier that the parasympathetic system is closely related to the yin component of the body, and the sympathetic to the yang component. Therefore, kidney yin deficiency corresponds, though it is not absolutely equivalent, to an inactive or suppressed parasympathetic nervous system, whereas the kidney yang deficient state corresponds to weakened sympathetic functions.

Patients with kidney deficiency of various reasons may be predominantly kidney yang deficient or kidney yin deficient, or they may be deficient in both. The second salient point about kidney deficiency syndromes is that this particular symptom complex is found in a wide variety of medical illnesses. By way of example, six disease categories, including bronchial asthma and anovulatory functional uterine bleeding, discoid or systemic lupus erythematosus, neurasthenia, which is equivalent to the modern day chronic fatigue syndrome, coronary atherosclerosis, and toxemia of pregnancy were studied, and each was found to share the same symptom complex of kidney deficiency in a traditional Chinese medical sense. These disease entities are listed in Key K-3 for reference.

<u>Some Clinical Entities of</u>
<u>Kidney Qi Deficiency</u>

- Bronchial asthma
- Anovulatory functional uterine bleeding
- Discoid or systemic lupus erythematosus
- Chronic fatigue syndrome
- Coronary atherosclerosis
- Toxemia of pregnancy

Although these are distinctly different disease entities from the viewpoint of modern medical science, the subjective symptoms and the objective physical findings including laboratory studies reveal that they share a number of common denominators rather typical of kidney deficiency syndromes in TCM. And as a practical matter, patients with these diagnoses were treated similarly with therapeutic medical agents in Chinese medicine known to tonify the kidney system and, lo and behold, the therapeutic efficacy was significantly superior to the available modern therapeutic regimens which included the use of steroids. The conclusion is that the singular tonification of the kidney system is effective in treating several diseases which are thought to be pathophysiologically different in terms of modern medical concepts.

Point #2 – The subjective symptoms of kidney deficiency can be correlated with objective physical and biochemical findings in the laboratory. The urine of these patients was collected in a 24 hour period. The amount of 17-hydroxycortical steroids contained in these samples was analyzed, and the results are summarized in Key K-4.

17 Hydroxycorticosteroids in 24 Hour Urine

Average in *Normal* subjects	**7.8 mg/24 hours**
Average in *Yin deficient* subjects	**6.5 mg/ 24 hours**
Average in subjects deficient in both Yin and Yang - but *predominantly Yin deficient*	**7.1 mg/ 24 hours**
Average in subjects *deficient in both kidney Yin and Yang*	**16.2 mg/ 24 hours**
Average in Subjects *deficient in kidney Yang*	**2.2 mg/ 24 hours**

In the normal subjects, the average was about 7.8 mg in a 24 hour period. The average in the yin deficient subjects was a little lower, 6.5 mg in 24 hours, whereas the average in subjects deficient in both yin and yang but predominantly yin deficient was 7.1 mg, not substantially different from the previous figures.

But here is the major deviation from normal: The average in subjects deficient in both kidney yin and yang was 16.2 mg per 24 hours. And then finally, in the subjects who were deficient in kidney yang, it was 2.2 mg per 24 hours.

As you can see, the two most notable findings in this experiment are that yang deficient individuals have a much lower content of 17-hydroxycorticosteroids in the urine, whereas individuals who are deficient in both yin and yang components have almost twice as much of this substance than normal, and we will try to explain why this is the case a little later.

Point #3 – The various kidney deficient states in the traditional Chinese medical sense also correlate well with the different patterns of the cold pressor test, which consists of immersing the hand of the experimental subject into 0 to 4 degree C ice water, and then taking systolic blood pressure readings at 30 seconds and 1 minute, then removing the hand from the ice water and continuing to take readings at 2 minutes, 5 minutes, 10 minutes and 15 minutes respectively. You may want to note here that cold immersion is considered a strong stress to the body. The cold immersion test is not only used to stress laboratory animals such as rats so that one may observe the physiological changes in many experiments studying the stress response, but this is in fact the prime screening test for Navy

SEALS. The Navy will make the enlistees go through a series of very rigorous trainings and then expose them to the very cold seawater near the Coronado Beach of San Diego. They get so cold that they may lose urine involuntarily and many enlistees drop out at this time because they can't stand the cold. As the saying goes, if you can't stand the heat, get out of the kitchen, and if you can't stand the cold, get out of the Navy SEALS.

So the stress of cold immersion, even of the hand alone, can cause the body to react strongly with a very clear-cut autonomic response which can be measured by a change in the blood pressure, particularly the systolic blood pressure. The shape of the blood pressure curve so obtained corresponded quite well to the different kidney deficiency states diagnosed from traditional clinical information alone. The results obtained are shown in Key K-5 and Key K-6.

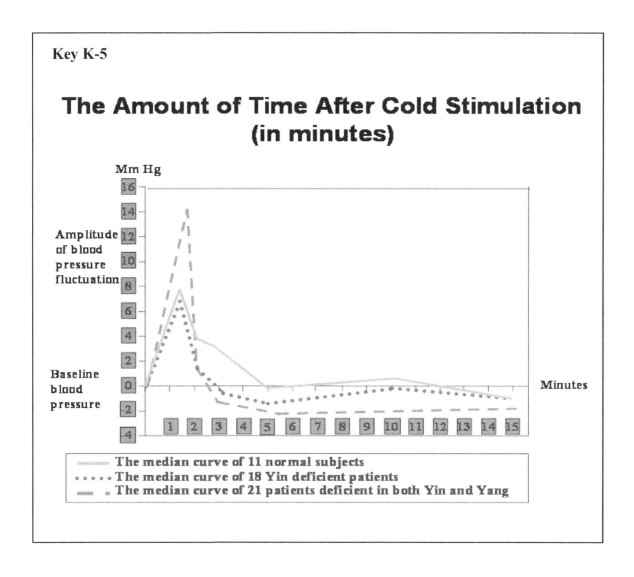

Key K-5

The Amount of Time After Cold Stimulation (in minutes)

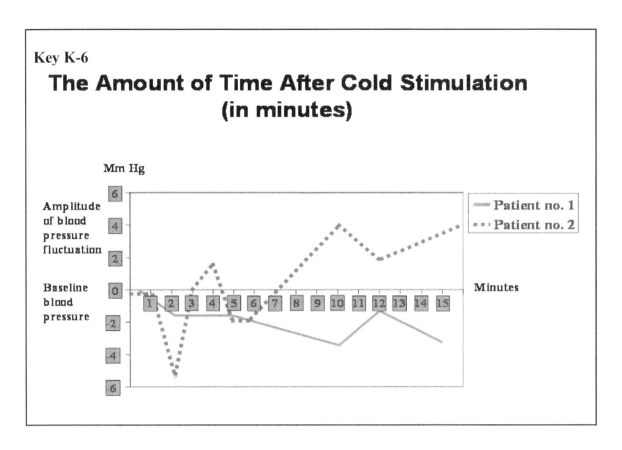

Key K-6

The Amount of Time After Cold Stimulation (in minutes)

Normal individuals responded to cold stimulus briskly but moderately, with the blood pressure returning to the normal level fairly quickly, requiring approximately 5 minutes. Primarily yin deficient subjects, however, responded equally briskly to the same stimulus, but their blood pressure quickly dropped below the baseline level, and it took approximately twice as long, or about 10 minutes for them to return to the baseline level. And individuals who are deficient in both yin and yang not only responded briskly to the stimulus, but also in an exaggerated manner, followed by a quick reversal by dropping below the baseline level and requiring a much longer period for full recovery to the baseline blood pressure. And finally, primarily yang deficient individuals reacted even more erratically to the cold stimulus, often with an initial decrease, rather than increase in blood pressure, which may then have been followed by a fluctuation above and below the baseline. See Key K-6.

Point #4 – The various kidney deficiency states can be rectified by the appropriate use of Chinese medical agents, including a number of herbal ingredients which can be classified as kidney yin or kidney yang tonifiers. With the institution of effective therapy, the biochemical indicators, such as the 24 hour urinary excretion of 17-hydroxy and 17-ketocorticosteroids, as well as objective physical parameters such as the cold pressor test curve can change hand-in-hand with the evolution of the kidney deficiency state. For instance, kidney tonifiers can convert a predominantly kidney yin deficient state into a predominantly kidney yang deficient state, as the yang component may now seem relatively weak when compared to a functionally augmented yin component. Sometimes the various kidney deficient states can also evolve into one another spontaneously, without intervention or therapy. In other words, a patient who is more yang deficient may suddenly become more yin deficient, or vice versa, with the accompanying sudden shifts in symptoms.

Summarizing all these points; the significance of the above data is the establishment of the validity of a seemingly abstract concept in TCM, by making it more tenable, and defining it with a series of biochemical parameters.

So this is very valuable information in assisting the diagnosis and treatment of diseases associated with the so-called kidney deficiency syndromes. Still, the symptom-complex of kidney deficiency and its associated clinical findings, together with their physiological mechanisms, continue to elude simple theoretical interpretations. For example, what is the explanation of the different patterns of cold pressor test curves associated with the different types of kidney deficiency states? And why would the 24 hour urinary excretion of 17 hydroxy or ketocorticosteroids in patients deficient in both kidney yin and kidney yang have twice as much as that of a normal person? Yet, kidney yang deficient individuals have a subnormal level. Furthermore, how can yin deficient states be so quickly transformed spontaneously into yang deficient states, and vice versa?

On the other hand, the clinical model following the traditional Chinese medical principles based on clinical symptoms alone is both simple and elegant, without resorting to elaborate knowledge in modern basic sciences. So it is essential to formulate a theoretical model which would take all these factors, as well as other related traditional Chinese medical principles, into account.

Here are my theoretical interpretations of the clinical and experimental findings:

1. First of all, the central nervous system is the cradle of a variety of diseases, or at the least it plays a vital role in mediating many pathophysiological processes not yet recognized by modern medicine. Traditional Chinese medical therapies deal directly with the CNS by modulating its functions, which in turn influences the disease processes. The reason TCM has been so difficult to be interpreted on the basis of modern medical sciences is because the central nervous system functions represented by traditional Chinese medicine are either undiscovered or poorly understood. But after we have realized the importance of the CNS, as we have discussed recently, we should be able to have a much clearer understanding of how the whole system works.

2. A hierarchy should exist within the CNS itself. In other words, not all parts of the brain are equal in terms of control. Now, we understand the brain controls many of the peripheral functions, but who is the master of the brain?

We think the ancient part of the brain which is close to the base of the brain, such as the hypothalamus or the thalamus, is the senior part of the brain, that in the course of evolution those structures were there first, before all the newer parts of the brain including the neocortex or the frontal cortex came into existence. They behave as if they are the roots of the brain, and they retain much control over the rest of the brain. This ancient brain is closely related to embryological development and is somehow closely linked to the urogenital system, which is closely linked to the autonomic nervous system, consisting of the sympathetic and the parasympathetic.

3. The central and peripheral neurons specializing in the parasympathetic functions can be considered the yin neurons of this system, whereas those specializing in the sympathetic functions can be considered the yang neurons.

4. In a state of health, the activities of the yin and yang neurons are not only balanced, but must also be adequate in amount of activities. To illustrate this point, let's take a look at a scale. If you put one marble on each side of the scale, the scale is balanced. If you put 10 marbles on each side, it is still balanced, but are these two balanced states identical? Most definitely not, and we'll see why.

A deficiency state of either yin or yang can be considered a result of either a decrease in the number of the functional neurons, or a decrease in their potency, or both. For simplicity's sake, the relative activity of either component can be expressed in what we can call neuronal units, which represent the equivalent potency of one single normally functioning yin or yang neuron. So, one unit of neuronal activity can be accomplished if you have two neurons each functioning at half capacity. Or if 50% of the neurons are working normally while the other 50% are non-functioning, you will also have a system that is half as efficient as normal.

5. The progression of disease usually follows a general pattern. When stress, whether physical or emotional takes place, the body will react in the following manner. First: Before the stress occurs or shortly afterwards, there is a normal amount of yin and yang that is followed by an excess of yang and a deficiency of yin, followed then by deficiency of yin and yang, and finally resulting in further deficiency of yin and still greater deficiency of yang. This pattern is illustrated in Key K-7. We'll come back to this diagram in a future discussion.

Key K-7

Health = Balance of Yin and Yang

1. CNS Controls Peripheral Functions

2. CNS Controls Via → | Autonomic Nervous System |

| CNS Yang Neurons | | CNS Yin Neurons |

Sympathetic   Parasympathetic

3. Strength of Yang = Number of Yang Neurons x Potency of Yang Neurons
   Strength of Yin = Number of Yin Neurons x Potency of Yin Neurons

4. Kidney Yin and Kidney Yang = A Biological Buffer System

---

6. The kidney concept. One must be careful not to confuse the kidney concept or kidney deficiency concept with the physical kidneys themselves, although there still exists a relatively close relationship. When we talk about the kidney deficiency concept, we are not talking about just the renal functions. The patient may not have a decrease in, say, 24 hour creatinine clearance. There may not be any problems with renal blood flow; there may not be any problem with kidney stones. The kidney concept in traditional Chinese medicine is far more inclusive. It encompasses not only the entire urogenital system, but also the adrenal gland, which is functionally and embryologically a part of the sympathetic outflow, as well as a number of CNS functions, including the emotion fear, and the faculty of hearing. We will delve deeper into this area during the face-to-face sessions, when we examine the five elements and the concepts of organ phenomena.

Now equipped with these understandings, we can proceed to explain some of the phenomena we observed in association with kidney deficiency syndromes, including the cold pressor test results, the pattern of the 17-hydroxy and 17 ketocorticosteroids in urine, and the associated symptomatology.

Now the first principle: The kidney yin and kidney yang together act as a buffering system, maintaining the homeostasis of the body.

Since it has been repeatedly emphasized in traditional Chinese medicine that the balance of yin and yang forces of the body must be maintained in order to achieve good health, a great deal of emphasis has been placed on the relative amount of yin and yang, but not quite enough attention has been paid to the absolute quantity of yin and yang, regardless of whether they are balanced are not. As we have just pointed out, the amount of yin and yang, or parasympathetic and sympathetic activities, depend on the number of yin and yang neuronal units, whether peripheral or central, that are operative at any one time. Yin and yang forces of the body can remain in balance at a given moment, whether the absolute amount of each is small or large, as long as they are equal. As in the example of marbles on the scale we cited earlier, this concept is also illustrated in Key K-8. These two different states, although balanced, are markedly different in terms of their stability. If there are an abundant number of operative neuronal units in both the yin and yang systems, any given amount of change will tip the balance only slightly, as the change represents only a small fraction of the total yin and yang available. The ratio between the neuronal units of the yin and yang compartments remains close to 1.

However, the same amount of change in an individual with substantially fewer operative yin and yang neuronal units – let's say he or she is deficient in both yin and yang – although balanced at the outset, will produce a major shift in the balance, as this same change now constitutes a much larger fraction of the original yin and yang available. The ratio of yin and yang in this case deviates significantly from 1, or as in the case of the scale, it swings widely, and symptoms of either yin deficiency or yang deficiency will quickly ensue (Please refer to Key K-8).

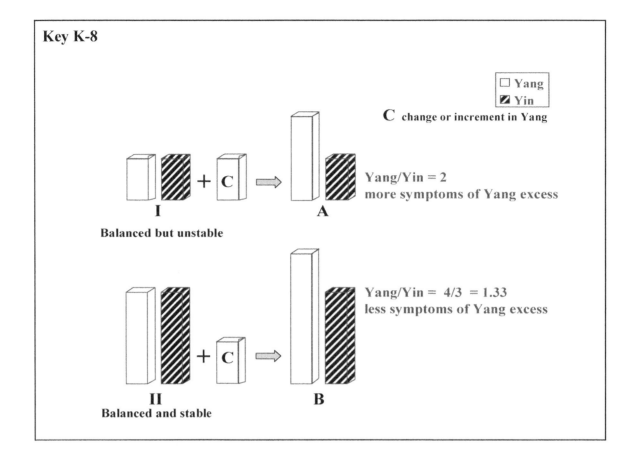

Key K-8

Yang
Yin

C change or increment in Yang

I
Balanced but unstable

A

Yang/Yin = 2
more symptoms of Yang excess

II
Balanced and stable

B

Yang/Yin = 4/3 = 1.33
less symptoms of Yang excess

As a result, the greater the amount of yin and yang or the greater the number of neuronal units operative before any change induced by stress takes place, the more stable the system and the more likely a harmonious internal environment can be maintained. So as in Key K-7, where you find tall bars in both yin and yang, that particular individual is extremely healthy. This is Clark Kent, Superman, or Wonder Woman, as these individuals just don't get sick easily, no matter what kind of stress you subject them to. They just bounce right back.

The properties of such a system are not unlike those of the acid-base buffering solution. The reason it is a buffer is that whether you add acid or base to this solution, the pH will not suddenly change, and obviously such a buffer system is advantageous to maintaining homeostasis in a biological system. This yin and yang buffering system will prevent the organism from deviating from normal very much at any one time. To carry this inference further, a patient with yin deficiency symptoms but who still has a good supply of yin and yang neuronal units is actually more stable and healthier than one who is for the moment asymptomatic due to a balanced but deficient yin and yang.

In this latter case of deficiency of both yin and yang, the balanced state will not last very long. Because it is so very unstable, either symptoms of yin excess or yang excess -- or if you want to put it another way, either symptoms of yin deficiency or yang deficiency -- will soon evolve and become apparent.

It has been the common experience of traditional Chinese medical practitioners that certain debilitated individuals who have a much reduced reserve of the total body yin and yang are the most difficult to treat because if you give such a patient a good dose of a yin tonifier, he will quickly appear yang deficient. If you give him an average dose of a yang tonifier, he will become yin deficient. As his internal environment is highly unstable and extremely sensitive to change, foods and drugs can initiate these changes, but so can the environment, as well as emotional changes. The body will tend to vacillate between the yin and yang directions.

Many patients with severe deficiency of both yin and yang can easily go through a series of erratic fluctuations from yang excessive to yin excessive symptoms, induced by the slightest change in the diet, which may contain yin or yang substances, or in association with environmental changes, such as the passing of a cold or warm front. Clinically the absolute yang and yin concept proposed here may be quite relevant. For example, a patient who is prone to inflammation or symptomatology of yang excess may in fact be deficient of both yin and yang, but with a greater deficiency of yin energy. A therapeutic regimen may be erroneously geared towards suppressing the yang component, producing further decrement of the yang, resulting in temporary relief of the symptoms of relative yang excess, but quickly followed by exacerbation because the system is now even more unstable, and complications can set in very quickly.

Consequently, the absolute amount of yin and yang, or the total yin and yang neuronal activities, must be estimated in addition to the relative activities of the two forces, when you are clinically assessing a patient.

The second important point about the physiological basis of these yin and yang deficiency states is that they are often markers for the manifestations of the different stages of the evolution of diseases, particularly diseases involving a degenerative process.

Approximately 1800 years ago, during the Han dynasty, a towering figure in the history of traditional Chinese medicine by the name of Zhang Zhongjing wrote the book *Shang Han Lun,* the direct translation of which is Cold Injury Thesis.

Superficially the title means the study of diseases originating from exposure to cold, such as catching a cold or getting an upper respiratory infection. In substance, however, this very book may be considered the bible of herbal medicine. It details the diagnosis and treatment of essentially all infectious diseases, and carefully describes the evolution from one syndrome to another, detailing the progression through the different phases of diseases.

The general pathway of progression is from the exterior towards the interior of the body. The outermost layer of the body is usually the first to be affected, and gives rise to a particular set of symptomatology, known in TCM as the greater yang or Tai Yang syndrome. As we progress through the different learning phases of this course, we will encounter in more detail the treatment of this subject. So for the purpose of the present discussion, we can simply say that the progression moves from the three layers of the exterior to the three layers of the interior, or from the yang to the yin. Although the disease may affect more than one division or one layer at any one time, and may progress rapidly from one division to another, or may even skip a certain division, this general rule holds true. From the modern medical standpoint, this rule can be interpreted to mean that lines of defense controlled by the central nervous system give way one-by-one following a particular order, and the involvement of each particular layer or division is associated with a particular, specific syndrome consisting of a definite set of symptoms and physical findings.

When the body is subject to either physical or emotional stress induced by infective agents or chemical insults, or physical traumas or anything else, the body in conjunction with the central nervous system responds by reacting to these insults by mobilizing the healing power of the body.

The first stage of such a response is usually inflammatory, corresponding to a state of yang excess. As the yang component dominates, the yin forces will be concomitantly suppressed, resulting in a yin deficient-yang excessive state. After this acute phase of response is over, if demand is continuously made upon these yin and yang neurons which are members of both the central and peripheral autonomic nervous systems, to cope with the external or internal environmental stresses, it tends to deplete the neurotransmitters of these neuronal units, and also their cellular reserves. We of course do not know yet what these reserves are made of, maybe proteins; maybe peptides; maybe other types of chemicals including messenger RNAs, or the products of other gene expressions.

This process will lead to a sub-acute phase, with deficiency of both the yin and yang components, with the yang components more likely to remain relatively excessive. As the pathological reactions wear on, the yang component consisting of the yang neuronal units is more reactive and therefore depletes faster than the yin section. Finally, in the advanced chronic stage, both yin and yang are further depleted, only this time the yang component becomes more deficient.

In accordance with the *Nei-Jing,* the Yellow Emperor's Classic on Internal Medicine, the nature of the yang element is expansive and reactive, whereas the yin qi is conservative, sustaining and less reactive.

Such a concept is in excellent agreement with known functions of the sympathetic and parasympathetic systems. The sympathetic nervous system is activated in fight or flight, and of course needs to be quickly responsive. The parasympathetic functions or yin functions tend to be activated at the time of safety, during which rest, digestion and other biological functions of sustenance usually take place. The sympathetic nervous system expends energy, whereas the parasympathetic nervous system conserves it. Consequently, it is reasonable that the sympathetic system or the yang component is more quickly reactive and can also be inactivated more readily than the yin components. It is also reasonable that yang forces tend to react first. The slower reacting yin functions also tend to be the last to be depleted. As a result, the following chain of biological events is often encountered in the progression of disease or in the deterioration of health, as in many degenerative processes. Now refer to Key K-9.

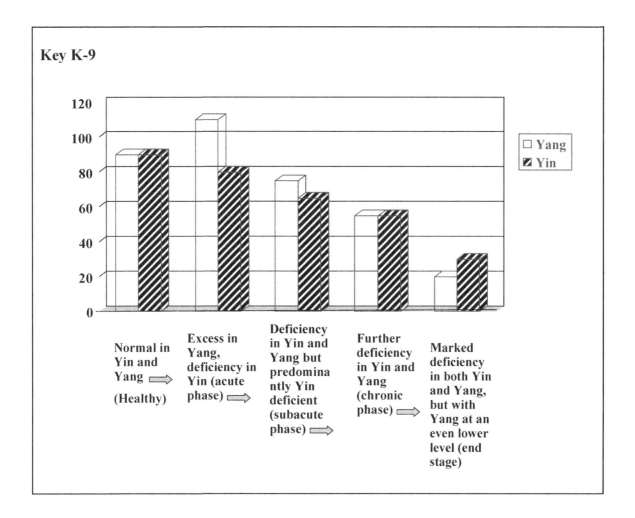

Key K-9

First we start out with normal yin and yang. When the body is stressed, the yang force becomes reactive, so there is a yang excessive state accompanied by a yin deficiency. But at this early stage, both the absolute amount of yin and the absolute amount of yang are relatively close to the normal level. When the disease process continues, however, as the body spends more energy on yang, it has to rely on yin to generate more yang energy, so both systems will begin to deplete. But yang is still the prime force or reaction, so it remains relatively excessive. The continuous expenditure of energy in both the yin and yang systems will eventually lead to a depletion of both yin and yang. And finally, when both systems are exhausted by the degenerative process, there is a state of extreme depletion of both yin and yang – except in this case, since yang is usually the reactive force, it is obvious that the yang is not capable of reacting anymore, and therefore it is apparently more deficient than yin.

Hans Selye, the very famous researcher in physiology based at McGill University of Canada, elegantly demonstrated experimentally that different phases follow an excess of stress. He was the one who proposed that mild stress is beneficial for the body because it stimulates the body, whereas severe stress -- in other words, stress that is beyond the ability of the organism to cope -- becomes distress.

In his model there is at first, alarm, and the body responds to the stress by adaptation, by mobilizing its resources. And if the stress becomes overwhelming, the body will finally reach an exhausted state, with derangement of its various organic systems. Although Dr. Selye emphasized more the endocrine functions' roles in coping with stresses whereas the dynamic proposed here concerns itself mainly with the nervous system, particularly the central nervous system, the fundamental pathophysiological basis may indeed be the same. For scientific evidence is ample that the nervous system and the endocrine system are basically inseparable in accomplishing any physiological purpose. The hypothalamus actually sends signals through nerves into the pituitary to secrete hormones, and hormones often interact with nerve tissues. So, one can think of the hormones as a mobile nervous system that can be circulated in the bloodstream to the target organs or tissues. The 17-hydroxy and 17-ketocorticosteroids are the metabolic products of steroids of the adrenal gland, and we have shown that these are closely related to the yin and yang deficiency states. So when the body is overstressed, it will no longer be able to respond to further stress, and therefore the extreme kidney deficiency state has been reached.

In the type II diabetic, the problem is with insulin resistance. The same amount of insulin is no longer effective in doing the job, so the problem may be related to the muscles. And forcing the pancreatic cells to work harder to release more insulin is not really the answer. It's like a horse that is galloping as fast it can, but then you whip it to make it go even faster and what happens is ultimately you exhaust the horse. It might even drop dead on you, and this is exactly what we are doing while we use sulfonylurea in the treatment of type II diabetes.

As you recall in the subjects who are deficient in both yin and yang, the 17-hydroxycorticosteroid level in the urine is twice as high as normal. In patients with advanced congestive heart failure, the circulating catecholamines are also found to be much more elevated than normal, and both the 17-hydroxycorticosteroids and catecholamines are products related directly to the adrenal gland, or the adrenal axis, which has a lot to do with stress. So these patients are literally stressed out, and it's little wonder why these patients with a high level of circulating catecholamines will have a much higher mortality rate than those who do not have an elevated level. As these patients have already reached a very advanced level of kidney qi deficiency in both yin and yang, we see that the principles of traditional Chinese medicine really have excellent correlation with modern medical science. And I can assure you: With the passing of time, the TCM principles will be widely accepted by modern medicine, and will do much to further the understanding of how the body works, and how diseases get generated.

Now let's take a moment to revisit the theoretical dispute between Dr. Zhu Danxi and Dr. Zhang Jing Yueh. Remember the former said that yang is often excessive and yin is often deficient while the latter said yang is never excessive and yin is often deficient? Well, using our theoretical model, we can explain why they disagreed, and why in fact they did not disagree. They were just emphasizing different aspects of this yin and yang balance equation. Both were correct, but each refers to a different point on the yin-yang depletion continuum.

The early phases of disease often manifest themselves in a yang excessive state because yang is the force that reacts first and as the disease progresses, it shows signs of yin deficiency, which is why Dr. Zhu said yang is often excessive and yin is frequently deficient. Dr. Zhang, on the other hand, thought that the total amount of yin and yang in a human body is rather limited, so yin and yang will be deficient as the disease progresses. And as far as the total amount of yin is concerned, the more the merrier, because then the body is capable of fending off the assault by diseases or pathogens. And this is the reason he claimed that one can never have too much yin and yang -- because both tend to be deficient, especially in the end stage of development of the degenerative process. They were basically talking about different angles of the same problem; they did not fundamentally disagree with each other.

These are indeed very useful concepts because time and time again, you are going to run into various clinical situations when you may be stumped by what you observe. Is this patient suffering from yin deficiency or yang deficiency? Or both? And why do they suddenly become yin deficient when only yesterday they were yang deficient? Again, the concept of the buffer is extremely useful. There may be practitioners out there who spent years studying and practicing TCM without a clear understanding of this very concept. I was one of them before I overcame the theoretical hurdle and in a matter of minutes, you have received the answer to the puzzle which you have not yet even seen in its entirety. So I sincerely hope you will put this concept into good use in the future.

The third area of usefulness of our current concept is the interpretation of the results of the cold pressor test. In a normal individual, the functioning neurons in both the yin and yang segments are normal in activity and abundant in number. When a cold stimulus is induced, it constitutes an environmental stressor. The yang or sympathetic component will be the first to respond. The smooth muscles of the arterioles contract and the blood pressure rises briskly, and this is a natural response. Then the yin, or parasympathetic component, is a little more sluggish to respond, but soon catches up, and blood pressure drops back down to the baseline level.

The solid line representing the 11 normal subjects in Key K-5 is typical of this response: A brisk rise in blood pressure, and then it stabilizes, also very quickly. In the case of yin deficiency, although it is assumed that the absolute number of neuronal units in both the yang and yin components is subnormal, the blood pressure reacted more or less the same way as in the normal subjects, followed by an earlier drop to baseline level, and requiring a longer period to recover. This curve is represented by the solid line representing the average of 18 yin deficient patients, in Key K-5 also.

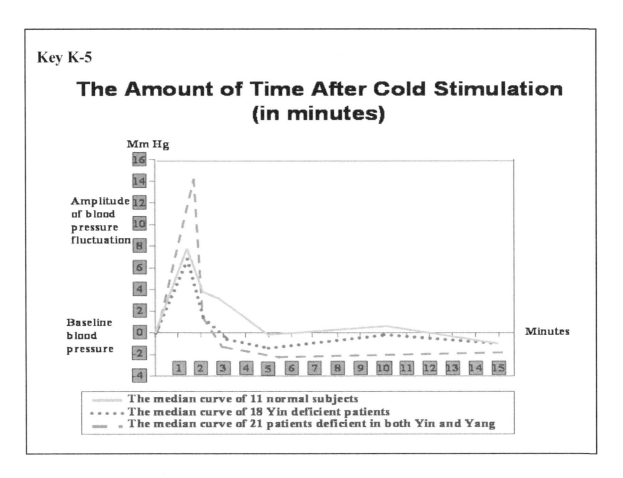

The Amount of Time After Cold Stimulation (in minutes)

Mm Hg

Amplitude of blood pressure fluctuation

Baseline blood pressure

Minutes

——— The median curve of 11 normal subjects
• • • • • The median curve of 18 Yin deficient patients
—— ▪ The median curve of 21 patients deficient in both Yin and Yang

The total duration of the positive deflection of the blood pressure curve seems to be determined by the number of yang neuronal units, which are now fewer in number due to some depletion as a result of disease. The fewer the yang neuronal units, the sooner the blood pressure will begin to fall, which is apparent from this diagram. Intuitively, we might expect the amplitude of the blood pressure rise to be less than normal because there are now fewer yang neurons, but in reality it is approximately equal to that of the normal subjects. The explanation is that the would-be reduced amplitude can easily be compensated by the decreased buffering capacity of the depleted yin and yang components, so that the expected lower peak of blood pressure rise is again exaggerated by this lack of control. So it winds up at the same spot as the normal subject. In this type of patient, the yin component is also less active. So the activation of the yin component which is responsible for dropping the blood pressure below baseline appears to take place later than in the normal subject, and is also more sluggish in returning to its normal activity. So you see, the curve drops down below baseline and then slowly recovers to the normal level.

Finally, in the case of a simultaneous yin and yang deficiency state, the response of the rise of blood pressure is exaggerated in magnitude, but it drops to baseline level earlier and remains so for a much longer period of time. According to our theoretical framework, the yin-yang deficiency state represents an even greater depletion of both components compared to the normal and the primarily yin deficient individuals. So the buffering capacity of the yin-yang system is further reduced, and the same cold stimulus causes a proportionally greater discrepancy between the yin and yang activities in the arterioles, producing greater constriction, and resulting in a greater rise of blood pressure. But due to fewer yang neuronal units, duration of the blood pressure rise is proportionally shortened. Here again, the deficient yin neurons behave more sluggishly, requiring an even longer period to recover to their normal degree of activity. As a result, the blood pressure remains below baseline level for a long time.

So the blood pressure curve from the cold pressor test of those individuals suffering from the simultaneously deficient yin and yang components appears to be an exaggeration of the curve of those individuals with yin deficiency.

You might want to think of the yin deficient state as being actually deficient of both yin and yang but more deficient in yin, whereas the simultaneous yin-yang deficiency represents a more advanced stage of deterioration of the yin and yang. They are more different in terms of quantity than quality.

From the above data, it seems that the amplitude of the rise of blood pressure depends on the buffering capacity of the yin and yang components, or in other words, it depends on the absolute number of the yin and yang neurons. The more depleted the yin and yang systems, the less ability they will have to buffer the change, and the more exaggerated the magnitude of response. The duration of the blood pressure rise, however, depends on the absolute potency of the yang component alone. The less potent it is, the shorter its duration of action. On the other hand, the less potent the yin neurons, the more sluggish they are in their response to the same stress. And once reacted, it takes them longer to recover their normal state of activity. This relatively simple model of progressive depletion of the yin and yang neuronal systems is quite consistent with experimental findings so far discussed.

Lastly, in the case of extreme depletion with the yang component at its lowest limit, the cold pressor test curve not only does not show any initial rise in blood pressure, but rather a reversal, which may even be followed by up and down fluctuations above the baseline in the course of time (refer to Key K-5 again). The lack of rise in blood pressure may indicate that the yang neurons are so exhausted or depleted of their cellular transmitters that their reactivity is abnormally delayed. The yin component, on the other hand, then has begun to respond after a latency period, resulting in a lowering of blood pressure. At this stage, the overall yin-yang system has deteriorated sufficiently to make the reactions unpredictable, and this corresponds to the advanced stage of a disease process which may be called the burnt out stage, or the end stage.

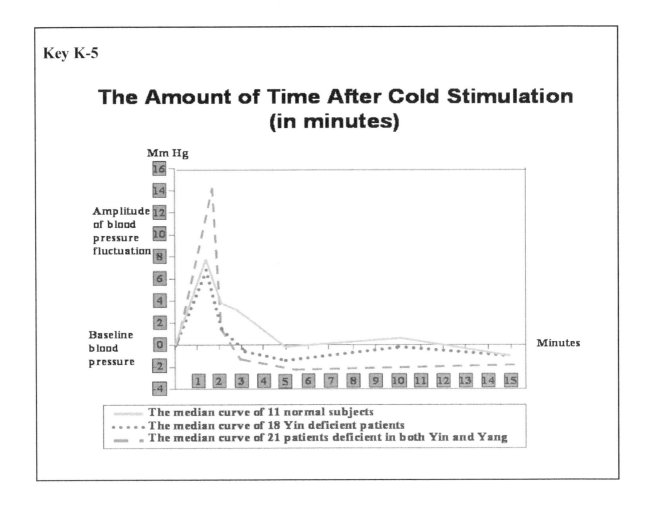

Key K-5

The Amount of Time After Cold Stimulation (in minutes)

Mm Hg

Amplitude of blood pressure fluctuation

Baseline blood pressure

Minutes

The median curve of 11 normal subjects
The median curve of 18 Yin deficient patients
The median curve of 21 patients deficient in both Yin and Yang

Now let's try to use this theoretical model to interpret biochemical findings in kidney deficiency syndromes. The cold pressor test is a very useful tool, however, it takes time to do, and you may have to train the staff to perform it just to find out whether the patient is yin deficient, yang deficient or deficient in both, and frankly, I don't know how you are going to get reimbursed for your time for doing this test. So its usefulness may be limited to a research setting, but this is not the case with lab studies such as testing the 24 hour urine **for** 17-hydroxy or 17-ketocortiosteroids, because these values are also highly useful in the evaluation of the patient as far as kidney qi deficiency is concerned. Here again, I would like to refer you to Key K-4.

In a small series of patients, the 24 hour urinary excretion of 17-hydroxycorticosteroids in yin deficient subjects was found to be quite close to the normal value. In the yin-yang deficiency state, however, the 17-hydroxycorticosteroids in the urine sharply increase to almost twice as much as normal, but the value quickly drops down to a very low level in the yang deficient state. So yin-yang deficiency probably corresponds to the time when the body is attempting to mobilize its resources in dealing with the stress of disease, whereas the yang deficiency state represents a final stage of exhaustion with little reserve to mobilize or to react with. Again, such data supports the hypothesis that the yin deficiency state is close to normal, with a yin-yang deficiency state being less normal, and the yang deficiency state least normal following the pattern of progression of diseases exactly.

Now the last application of our model is to attempt to explain other traditional Chinese medical principles, in association with the kidney deficiency concept.

Armed with this theoretical and actually very practical framework, we will now try to explain some of the enigmas in traditional Chinese medicine that are embodied in the kidney deficiency concept. This model is not only useful to explain the experimental data as well as a whole host of complex clinical problems, but it will also shed great light on a number of traditional Chinese medical principles related to the kidney system.

Health ought to be defined as the ability of the body to cope with stresses and changes in the environment, both internal and external.

This ability depends on the capacity to mobilize the body's reserves to meet certain situational demands, and to maintain the body in a state of physiological equilibrium. The control of the forces of mobilization is believed to be resident in the central nervous system. The neurophysiological mechanisms of the master portion of the brain are therefore equivalent to the traditional Chinese medical concept of kidney qi, sometimes known also as "prime qi". In accordance with traditional teachings, this prime qi, or ability to maintain the internal environment, is relatively weaker in the very young and the very old, and strongest in mid-life. And this accounts for the susceptibility to various diseases of the very young and the very old. So tonifying the kidney system is equivalent to regulating the controlling parts of the brain, thereby increasing the body's own ability to forestall further deterioration of the disease, or even reverse it. It is for this reason that tonification of the kidney system alone can have great beneficial effects on diverse types of diseases; this observation has been confirmed by other researchers in TCM, by way of clinical investigation.

Tonification, a term often used in traditional Chinese medicine, is a way to fortify the functions of the body. Tonification probably takes place in the controlling parts of the brain such as the hypothalamus and the thalamus which initiate a chain of physiological events peripherally. As we have said earlier, catecholamines and cortical steroids are hormones that cope with stress. They are the products of the adrenal gland, which in turn is controlled by the hypothalamus. So according to our hypothesis, this is, in fact, a part of the kidney system, the kidney system in the TCM sense, not in the modern anatomical sense. There is little wonder why steroids can be used to treat such a wide spectrum of clinical disorders such as asthma, rheumatoid arthritis, systemic lupus, idiopathic thrombocytopenia purpura, neoplasms, skin diseases of all types, and many other clinical disorders. In fact, if you take away steroids from dermatologists, they probably will lose half of their practice, if not more. And if steroids were no longer allowed in modern medicine, it would have a devastating effect on the management of chronic diseases.

Chapter Eight – Kidney Deficiency and Its Clinical Applications

Despite the extensive use of steroids such as Prednisone, Cortisone, Solu-Medrol, etc. in the treatment of a large variety of clinical disorders in modern medicine, and despite the fact that steroids are closely related to the urogenital system or the kidney system, because they are products of the adrenal gland, they represent only a part of this kidney system according to TCM, and are mainly peripheral vehicles or messengers. The central neuronal derangement, which is the basis of many disease states, often remains unchanged despite the use of steroids. And the usefulness of steroid therapy is often limited, as they only suppress symptoms, not necessarily changing the course of the disease.

Nonetheless, the tremendous therapeutic efficacy and the versatility of such products attest to the very concept of the kidney system in Chinese medicine, and though many of our colleagues have no knowledge of TCM, they actually use fundamental tenets of TCM when employing steroids to globally tonify the kidney system to treat a multitude of diseases. However, steroids may not be beneficial in all medical conditions; in fact they may be outright harmful in some situations. Even for the same clinical disorder, steroids may not be good for all patients. Why? Because these patients may have a predominantly yin deficient syndrome or a primarily yang deficient syndrome, or they may have deficiency in either system. Therefore, their response to steroids may vary, just like their metabolism of adrenal hormones may vary, as we have shown earlier, as reflected in the concentration of the 17-hydroxy and ketocorticosteroids excretion.

With the incorporation of TCM into the mainstream of western medicine, on the other hand, traditional Chinese medical therapy can be titrated to suit the individual patient's needs. Its therapeutic actions, instead of mainly focusing on peripheral functions, are most likely mediated by central mechanisms, and therefore are much more effective in changing or reversing the clinical course of the disease, accomplishing what is known as long-term cure.

Another important concept relating to the kidney deficiency syndrome is that the kidney system relates primarily to the "essence", the fundamental material that the kidney system is said to govern, build and store, and which carries our most foundational information through our lives and through our descendants. We will cover more about essence in this section.

Ancient Chinese physicians considered the kidney system to be the reservoir of essence, and that it can be converted to qi or energy. On the surface, this concept may seem inexplicable. However, if one equates qi with neural transmissions or the conduction of neural impulses, then essence may be equivalent to the biochemical compounds that produce such transmissions, namely the different types of neurotransmitters, their precursors or cellular organelles, or substances such as messenger RNAs, special proteins, peptides or cytokines or, in fact, whatever controls the biological mechanisms for its synthesis, which may include the genetic material within the neurons of the CNS.

In recent years, a lot of research has been done on the treatment for congestive heart failure using two important classes of drugs: beta-blockers and ACE inhibitors. These two medications not only improve the functional capacity of the patients, decreasing their symptoms, but more importantly, prolong their lives. Nobody really knows exactly how they accomplish this unusual feat. Patients who are suffering from congestive heart failure are also found to have increased circulating catecholamines such as norepinephrine, and in fact, if the level exceeds 600 picogram, the mortality of this group of patients increases dramatically. These are the recently observed, very intriguing clinical phenomena in modern medicine.

Now, how do we put all these data into the proper perspective?

I would like to note at this point that with the minimal amount of knowledge you have just acquired, you have already built a sufficient theoretical framework to solve some of the mysteries we have just mentioned.

Referring back to Key K -4, you note that in subjects deficient in both kidney yin and yang, the average of the 17-hydroxycorticosteroids in the urine in 24 hours is 16.2 mg. This is more than twice normal. The body at this stage is pouring out stress hormones because the body senses that the crisis is ongoing, so something has to be done about it, therefore it keeps on reacting by turning out all these neural hormones. The circulating catecholamines in advanced congestive heart failure patients are equally indicative of the yin and yang deficiency state.

Key K-4

<u>17 Hydroxycorticosteroids in 24 Hour Urine</u>

Average in *Normal* subjects	**7.8 mg/24 hours**
Average in *Yin deficient* subjects	**6.5 mg/ 24 hours**
Average in subjects deficient in both Yin and Yang - but *predominantly Yin deficient*	**7.1 mg/ 24 hours**
Average in subjects *deficient in both kidney Yin and Yang*	**16.2 mg/ 24 hours**
Average in Subjects *deficient in kidney Yang*	**2.2 mg/ 24 hours**

And the more desperately the body is trying to solve this alarming situation by turning on these neurohormonal mechanisms, the more energy it is going to spend, in this case the yang energy.

And since yang energy is a derivative of yin energy and qi is a product of essence, the more yang energy or qi the body mobilizes, the more energy it will expend, and the faster it will deplete this vital resource. And when this vital energy source is exhausted, the patient cannot survive.

This explains why a patient with congestive heart failure with a high blood level of catecholamines actually will have increased mortality. Both beta-blockers and ACE inhibitors are yin substances: They are anti-yang drugs. And they are capable of toning down the sympathetic activities -- in other words, they are sympatholytic. Somehow they prevent the body from turning on this alarm system and prevent it from mobilizing the body's vital resources in a futile attempt to correct the underlying abnormalities.

The essence or jing, in Chinese, behaves like a bank deposit. The faster you make withdrawals, the sooner the account balance will dwindle, and the sooner the check is going to bounce. So preventing withdrawals from this account will ensure the balance will last longer. Interestingly, the behavior of yin and yang in the biological system is quite similar to the behavior of energy and mass in the physical world. To explain this parallel, Einstein's famous equation "$E = MC^2$" comes in quite handy. E, of course, stands for energy, M for mass, and C for the speed of light. Since C is a very large number and C^2 is even larger, a little bit of mass is equivalent to a lot of energy, and that is of course the working principle of the atom bomb. What Einstein told us is that mass can be converted into energy, and energy to mass. Energy and mass are nothing more than different expressions of the same thing. So think of mass as concentrated energy and energy as dispersed mass.

In TCM, yang is energy, Yin is substance, or mass, or essence. So when yin is consumed and dispersed, it becomes yang and when yang is concentrated, it becomes yin. They are in fact mutually convertible.

In an acute illness such as an infection, yang is first mobilized, and this expenditure of yang energy has to come from somewhere, namely the yin or the essence. So when a fever continues or the stress continues, yang is being consumed, and indirectly yin will have to ultimately pay the price by supplying the yang with its substances or essence.

So as the disease advances, both yin and yang will be depleted.

According to TCM, the so-called essence is limited in supply, and will become depleted in the course of time, resulting in a gradual waning of qi, which can account for the process of aging. In a situation where the demand on the mobilization of qi is great, or for a prolonged period of time, premature depletion of these neurotransmitters or yin substances or essence or qi will take place. Damage may be imposed on the controlling cellular mechanisms due to the overburden, leading to premature deterioration of qi or vital energy as a result. The ability to cope with stress is compromised, and diseases will soon ensue. It is maintained in traditional Chinese medicine that excessive use of physical strength, overexertion, trauma, extreme emotions -- especially the emotion fear -- can also produce kidney deficiency as a syndrome. The common denominator here is excessive mobilization or taxing of the controlling neurons in the CNS for coping with stress. The emotion fear can produce more damage to this system because it primarily demands response from the sympathetic nervous system, which is a major component of the kidney yang system. Since we are going to discuss in some details about the kidney system within the context of the five elements concept later on, we are not going spend much time here now, but it is worthwhile mentioning that physical exertion commonly depletes the kidney qi. Case in point: Many trained women athletes develop amenorrhea as a result of their hard physical training. They stop menstruating because their kidney system has been weakened; it cannot conserve its energy enough to condition the body to be receptive to pregnancy. It is really the wisdom of the body saying, "Well, in the condition that you are in, I don't want you to get pregnant because you are physically not fit". Unfortunately, women athletes sometimes overtrain chronically, so they may get their gold medals, but what price must they pay?

Remember also Jim Fixx? The guru that is famous for his books on running? He died from a heart attack during one of his runs! So it's clear from the teachings of TCM that excessive exercise is actually detrimental to one's health.

Another maxim of traditional Chinese medicine states that "Prolonged illness eventually involves the kidney system." Chronic illnesses impose a continuous and excessive workload on the mobilizing force of the CNS, causing it to fatigue and be depleted. So whatever the disease may be, it can lead to similar results physiologically."

As mentioned earlier, the final stage of disease usually ends up in a kidney yang deficiency state. This can be exemplified by so-called "burned out rheumatoid arthritis". After years of chronic illness of this nature, the signs of inflammation subside because there is very little yang energy that the body is left to react with. The early days of inflammation are equivalent to the yin deficiency state. Finally, as the urogenital system is closely related to this central controlling part of the brain, its functions often deteriorate in parallel with the central neuronal functional derangement. This is why kidney functions decrease with the increase of age. Creatinine clearance decreases, and BUN increases, a rather common laboratory finding in the aged.

The roles played by the central nervous system in the generation and the evolution of disease have been basically ignored in modern medicine, and it is for this very reason that it is characteristically less effective in coping with the large variety of chronic diseases, compared to traditional Chinese medical modalities. Since modern medicine deals primarily with the peripheral biochemical and physiological phenomena (peripheral in terms of being outside of the CNS), therapy is often based on suppression of symptoms. On the other hand, traditional Chinese medicine acts on the CNS directly, enabling the body to mobilize its own ability to reestablish an optimal milieu interior, or internal environment.

Now that we recognize that kidney deficiency can be found in so many disease states as a shared pathway of many pathological processes, let's take a look at a real life example of how the kidney deficiency concept can be applied in learning more about an individual disease entity. Let's use scleroderma as a prime example, to illustrate the concept of kidney deficiency. Scleroderma is of course one of the collagen diseases, and modern medical treatments are by and large ineffective, in most cases. According to TCM, scleroderma is rather typical of the kidney deficiency state with a penchant towards yang deficiency. According to our modern medical texts, incidence of scleroderma is about three times higher in women than in men, and the disease is much more severe and frequent in young black women. According to one study, the propensity for developing this disease is probably genetic in origin, because the normal incidence of this disease in the general population is from 19 to 75 per 100,000 individuals, whereas in the Choctaw Native American population in Oklahoma, the incidence is as high as 472 per 100,000, strongly suggestive of a genetic predisposition. According to TCM, women are generally more yin than men, and since scleroderma is a yin disease, which is also a different way of saying that it is a yang deficient disease, one will expect the incidence in women to be higher than it is in men. Also according to TCM, the color black belongs to the kidney system, which also represents the element water. So increased pigmentation is found in Addison's disease, the symptom complex of which is rather consistent with yang deficiency, and patients suffering from Addison's disease may also have increased skin pigmentation. And this may explain why in dark-skinned individuals, the disease of scleroderma or yang deficiency may be more severe. Scleroderma-like illnesses may also be precipitated by environmental factors.

In 1981, roughly 20,000 people in Spain after ingestion of adulterated rapeseed oil developed a multi-system disease very similar to scleroderma. Clinical findings included interstitial pneumonitis, eosinophilia, arthralgia, arthritis, myositis followed by joint contracture, skin thickening, Raynaud's phenomenon, pulmonary hypertension and resorption of distal fingertips, findings rather typical of scleroderma. And these findings are quite consistent with a yin system or a yang deficient system, often found in individuals with a cold constitution.

Jiang, Zhong, Guo and Chen, four investigators of the First Hospital of Shanghai, conducted a study using traditional Chinese medicine to treat patients suffering from scleroderma. They collected clinical data on seventeen cases of scleroderma, consisting of five males and 12 females. Six of the patients had skin manifestations only, and the 11 other patients had systemic manifestations.

The symptoms and signs of these patients with respect to kidney deficiency are outlined in the table, in Key K-10. Aside from the typical findings such as thickening of skin with loss of sensation, cold and cyanotic distal fingers, and limitation of motion in their joints, they also had symptoms of kidney deficiency of one type or another. For instance, tiredness and weakness of the lower back was found in 10 of these patients, weak extremities in four, heel pain in three, and ringing in the ears in five patients, loss of hearing in three, hair loss in six, teeth loosening in four, a weak proximal radial pulse in 16, and out of the 12 female patients, eight of them had menstrual irregularities.

111

Summary of Symptoms, Signs and Kidney Deficiency Types of 17 Cases of Scleroderma

Kidney Deficiency		Kidney Yang Deficiency		Kidney Yin Deficiency	
Symptoms:	# of Cases	Symptoms:	# of Cases	Symptoms:	# of Cases
Backache back tiredness	10	Aversion to cold & cold extremities	13	Dizziness	4
Weak extremities	4	Cold feeling on back	3	Visual disturbance	4
Heel pain	3			Small voiding of dark urine	2
Tinnitus	5	Spontaneous sweating	3	Constipation	3
Hearing loss	3	Preference for hot drinks	6	Insomnia	3
Premature greying of hair	1			Night sweat	5
		Sexual impotence	3	Nocturnal emission	1
Loose teeth	4	Decreased libido	1	Preference for cold drinks	1
Menstrual Irregularities	8	Numbness in extremities	8		
Signs		Large voidings of clear urine	3	**Signs**	
		Nocturia	3	Faint pulse	5
Weak chueh pulse (proximal radial pulse)	16	Pale or dusty Complexion	8	Soft or slippery pulse	4
				Bow pulse	2
		Signs		Tip + side of tongue red	2
		Pulse small & lax	6	Central fissures	3
		Bulky & delicate looking tongue	12	Central patches without coating	1
		Teeth marks	14		

Since they all suffered from kidney deficiency syndrome, you will find both the kidney yang deficient and kidney yin deficient symptoms, as listed in the two columns. But as you can see, the yang deficiency symptoms are more prominent. Thirteen of them not only had cold extremities, but they actually had strong aversion to a cold environment. Three of them even had a cold sensation in the back all the time. Since the back is of the yang domain, a lack of yang energy is particularly noticeable when there is a total lack of yang energy of the entire body. Three of them had spontaneous sweating. Sweating is usually a sign of excessive yang, but in this case there is a deficiency of both yin and yang, and yang is uncontrolled, indicating there is a more advanced state of kidney energy deficiency. Preference for hot drinks is usually a clear indication of internal cold, which can be ameliorated by putting hot fluids into the center of the body. Numbness in the extremities can occur because the yang energy does not travel to the distal portions of the limbs. If you hold onto an ice cube for a long time in your hand, your hand gets so cold that it gets numb. So numbness is oftentimes associated with a yang deficiency state. Some of these patients also suffered from frequency of urination and also nocturia, and the color of the urine tended to be clear, and the volume usually large. Spontaneous diuresis is usually indicative of a yang deficient state. Signs of yang deficiency will include a small or narrow pulse, a bulky and delicate looking tongue, teeth marks on the tongue due to excessive wetness in the system, as the teeth will make impression on the tongue because there is local edema. During the hands-on session in Phase 1, we will definitely revisit these diagnostic signs, as we touch upon the subjects of pulse diagnosis, tongue diagnosis, and diagnosis by history and physical examination.

You will also note in this table that yin deficiency symptoms also coexist in this syndrome, and sometimes you may see these symptoms sort of vacillate back and forth between the yin deficiency state and yang deficiency state. As we pointed out earlier, a more advanced degree of kidney deficiency will lead to a very unstable system because both the yin and yang components are weak, and therefore they have lost the ability to buffer, which is the ability to prevent the system from swinging from one extreme to the other, swinging from a yin deficient to a yang deficient manifestation. So some of the yin deficiency state symptoms such as night sweats, insomnia, constipation, nocturnal emission, dizziness and visual disturbances due to the pseudo-yang rising to the head, will also be found. Likewise, there could be some yin deficient physical signs, such as a slippery pulse or bow pulse (bow pulse is a very taut pulse, and we will explain that in the diagnostic session), or absence of, or patches of coating on the surface of the tongue.

Now let us turn our attention to an actual case study rather typical of the kidney deficiency state found in scleroderma. Please refer to Key K-11:

A Typical Case of Scleroderma

Chief Complaint: This 42 year old, married woman was admitted to the hospital due to pain and discoloration of her fingers for 16 years accompanied by hardening of skin and limitation of motions in her fingers for approximately 10 years.

History of Present Illness: In the month of October 16 years ago, patient suddenly experienced episodes of needlelike sharp pain in her fingers in association with a decrease of temperature in her hands along with fingers turning white and purple. These symptoms disappeared in February of the following year completely. During the subsequent years, the symptoms exacerbated during winter time and gradually disappeared in warmer weather. Twelve years ago, she noticed puffiness and swelling of her fingers without pitting. Ten years prior to admission the skin of her fingers began to harden, causing impairment of motion of her finger joints, resulting in an inability to make a fist together, with a numbing sensation at the tips of her fingers. Since the onset of these symptoms, she intermittently experienced a sensation of fatigue and weakness in her low back, ringing in the ear, dizziness, aversion to cold, preference for hot drinks, frequent dreams, insomnia and memory loss. Her menses stopped altogether 4 months ago. Various previous treatments at another hospital did not relieve her symptoms.

Physical Examination: A middle-aged woman who spoke with a low voice appeared to be chronically ill and emaciated. Facial expression was dull. Thinning of hair was apparent. The distal digits appear to be shortened. Skin on the fingers felt hard, thick and tight, with a wax like glossy appearance. There is a decrease of temperature in both hands with increased pigmentation. There was redness and tenderness at the tip of the right index finger. There was no limitation of extension of all the fingers but flexion was impaired and there was the inability to make a fist. Finger nails appeared to be dystrophic. Tongue was pale with teeth marks laterally and loss of coating centrally. The pulse was small and soft with weakness at the proximal positions.

Laboratory Findings: WBC 13,900 per mm^3, RBC 3,020,000 per mm^3, hemoglobin 11 gram percent, sedimentation rate 16 mm per hour, 24 hour urine 17 hydroxy corticosteroid 2.6 mg and 17-keto corticosteroid 5.2 mg. X-ray of both hands showed generalized bone thinning with bone resorption at proximal and distal ends of digits. Cold pressure test showed a paradoxical response. Urine and stool analyses were negative, electrophoresis, electrolytes, liver and kidney function tests and EKG were all unremarkable.

Diagnosis and Clinical Course: Western diagnosis was disseminated scleroderma and TCM clinical impression was kidney yang deficiency. The treatment plan was to tonify the kidney yang and mobilize the qi in the meridians using traditional herbal formulae. Eight days following admission, the patient felt she had regained some dexterity in her hands and the symptoms of low back weakness and tiredness, ringing in the ears, dizziness, insomnia and frequent dreams all had disappeared, although she was still complaining of aversion to cold, coldness of the extremities and her hands still turned purple when exposed to cold. The same therapeutic formula was continued for another 6 days and the patient's condition remained improved but unchanged from 6 days ago. The therapeutic formula was modified with the addition of ma huang, bei jia, jiang huang and hong hua. Another week later there appeared to be some softening of the skin in her digits with increased mobility and she could close her hands better than before. Aversion to cold and coldness in her extremities now had disappeared although the tongue appearance and the pulse characteristics remain the same. A new therapeutic formula based on the same diagnostic criteria was prescribed. Four days later on April 1, she noticed sweating in her hands whereas sweating was usually not noted until the beginning of June in previous years. The skin at the tip of her fingers was now much softer and she was able to make a complete fist. The therapeutic formula, once again modified with additions and subtractions of herbal ingredients was given to her for another 8 days before she was discharged. At the time of discharge, she had a pinkish complexion, her spirit was good, and there was marked reduction of the tightness of the skin enabling her to make a tight fist although there was still cyanotic reaction to cold exposure. The cold pressor test returned to normal on April 26 during an outpatient visit, when she was

A 42-year-old married woman was admitted to the hospital because of pain in her fingers, along with discoloration and hardening of the skin, and also limitation of motion of her fingers for the last 10 years or so.

History of present illness: In the month of October 16 years ago, the patient suddenly experienced an episode of needle-like sharp pain in her fingers, in association with a decrease of temperature in her hands, when her fingers would turn first white and then purple in color. As you well know, this history is quite consistent with Raynaud's phenomenon. About, 1/3 of patients present with Raynaud's phenomenon when they have scleroderma. According to TCM, patients with scleroderma have a cold constitution, and when the body is stressed by cold, either by cold environment or by touching a cold object such as reaching into the refrigerator and picking up an ice tray, it can precipitate these specific vasomotor responses in the peripheral part of their extremities. And these symptoms completely disappeared in February of the following year. In other words, the symptoms got worse during the winter months, and improved with the onset of spring. Twelve years ago, she noticed puffiness and swelling of her fingers without pitting. Non-pitting edema is typical of scleroderma. Ten years prior to admission, the skin of her fingers began to harden, causing impairment of the motion of her finger joints, causing her difficulties in making a fist, and there was a numbing sensation at the tips of her fingers.

It is worth remembering here that according to traditional Chinese medicine, many of the so-called arthritides, such as rheumatoid arthritis or gout, are caused by wetness and coldness and sometimes associated with so-called "wind syndrome". When the body gets cold, the qi flow begins to slow down, and the sensations of both pain and coldness can be perceived simultaneously. This lack of flow of energy also causes numbness.

Since the onset of these symptoms, she intermittently experienced a sensation of fatigue and weakness in her low back. The Chinese describe this sensation as sour or *suan*. I have difficulty in translating this term because there seems to be no exact equivalent in the English language concerning this sensation. *Suan* in Chinese sounds like sour, which is the exact feeling in a muscle when one tastes something very sour. This unpleasant sensation is, I guess, a kind of parasthesia, but it is a particular kind of unpleasant sensation and is not pain per se, and usually is associated with some degree of weakness and tiredness. She also suffered from ringing in the ears, dizziness, aversion to cold, preference for hot drinks, frequent dreams, insomnia and memory loss, all of which are manifestations of a kidney deficiency. Her menses stopped altogether four months earlier. When menstruation stops, you know that the underlying qi deficiency has gotten more severe. She was treated at a different hospital before, and the treatment was by and large ineffective.

Physical Examination: Patient appeared to be chronically ill, emaciated, and spoke with a low voice. A low voice because there is no internal energy, so the body tends to conserve energy by using as little qi or energy as possible. Facial expression was dull.

When the total body yang energy is depleted, the patient generally tends to be more depressed, and there is a decrease in psychomotor activities, which will lead to a lack of animation, thus her facial expression was dull. Thinning of hair was also apparent.

According to TCM, hair is the excess of kidney qi. In other words, only when one has an ample supply of kidney qi or energy will the hair grow to be shiny and healthy. So when the body's kidney qi is low, it has not enough energy to supply the vital organs, skin or the other parts of the body, so hair is the last thing the kidney will "think of", because hair is not as essential as other body parts for maintenance of vital functions. So looking at the condition of the hair, you can catch a glimpse of how well the body is doing, so the hair's condition often parallels the state of health.

The distal digits appeared to be shortened, skin on the fingers felt hard and thick and tight, with a wax-like glossy appearance. There was a decrease in temperature in both hands with increased pigmentation, and redness and tenderness at the tip of the right index finger was noted. Patient was able to extend all her fingers, but she had a hard time making a fist, and her fingernails appeared to be dystrophic. Tongue was pale with teeth marks laterally. This is a rather typical finding of yang deficiency, as we shall see during the tongue diagnosis session. And there was also a loss of coating in the central part of the tongue. The pulse was small and soft, with weakness at the proximal position. The proximal position represents the position of the kidney. So when the kidney is weak, this proximal pulse or the chueh pulse will also be weak.

Lab Findings: The WBC was almost 14,000; the RBC is just slightly over 3,000,000 and hemoglobin 11 g, substantially below normal. It's probably anemia due to chronic disease. The sed rate was 16 mm per hour and both the 17-hydroxycorticosteroids and 17-ketocorticosteroids were substantially below normal, at 2.6 mg and 5.2 mg respectively.

X-ray of both hands showed generalized bone thinning with bone resorption at proximal and distal ends of the digits, and here you should know a very interesting parallel between scleroderma and reflex sympathetic dystrophy, because both conditions are characterized by vasomotor instability, and a heightened sympathetic tone resulting in vasoconstriction is present in both of these clinical entities.

Additionally, the cold pressor test in this patient showed a paradoxical response which is rather typical of an advanced state of kidney deficiency. The balance of the lab findings including urinalysis, stool analysis, serum electrophoresis, electrolytes, liver and kidney function tests and EKG were all unremarkable. So the clinical impression according to TCM was kidney yang deficiency, and the treatment plan was to tonify the kidney yang and mobilize qi in the meridians, using traditional herbal medicine.

Some eight days following admission, the patient felt she had regained some dexterity in her hands, and the symptoms of low back weakness and tiredness, ringing in the ears, dizziness, insomnia and frequent dreams all disappeared after daily dosing of the kidney yang tonifiers. Although at this time she still complained of aversion to cold and objectively there was coldness in the extremities and Raynaud's phenomenon still persisted, as her hands still turned purple when exposed to cold. The same therapeutic formula was continued for another six days and the patient's condition remained about the same with no additional change. So the therapy was modified with the addition of *ma huang, bie jia, jiang huang* and *hong hua*, all different herbs in the Chinese therapeutic armamentarium. Another week later, there was softening of the skin in her fingers with increase in mobility and she was able to close her hands better than before. The aversion to cold and coldness in the extremities had now disappeared, although the tongue appearance and the pulse were the same as before. A new therapeutic formula based on the same diagnostic conclusion was prescribed. Four days later on April 1, she noticed she had sweating in her hands, though sweating was usually not noted until the beginning of June in previous years, anhydrosis is often found in patients suffering from scleroderma because of the disturbance in yang functions. The skin at the tip of her fingers was now much softer and she was now able to make a complete fist. The therapeutic formula was once again modified with addition and subtraction of herbs, and she received treatments for another eight days, whereupon she was discharged. At the time of discharge, she had a pinkish complexion and her spirit was lifted, and there was a marked reduction of the tightness of the skin, enabling her to make a tight fist. Her fingers, however, still reacted to cold with cyanosis.

About two weeks later on April 26 during an outpatient visit, she was found to have normal cold pressor test, and she had maintained all her clinical improvements. At that time, the WBCs were 8300 and RBCs had risen to 3.5 million approximately. Likewise, the 17-hydroxycorticosteroids and the 17-ketocorticosteroids per 24 hours had reached 8.7 mg and 9.35 mg respectively, substantially higher than the value on admission.

This particular case of study is quite instructive in several areas. It shows first that by a global management of the body by tonifying the kidney system, increasing the total body qi, significant improvements can be obtained even though the treatment itself may not be specific for that particular disease entity, in this case scleroderma. Secondly, when the patient's condition improves, both subjective symptoms and objective physical findings as well as lab findings will also improve in a parallel fashion, affirming the concept of kidney deficiency as something very real and not just imagined by the ancient physicians in China, even though they did not have any access to modern laboratory tools to follow the biochemical indices.

Yet they were able to accomplish a great deal using clinical information alone, as well as some of the rather primitive but highly effective techniques of diagnosis to accomplish the feat of healing in some ways still not matched by modern medical sciences.

While discussing scleroderma, I think it is worthwhile to mention a few points about Raynaud's phenomenon, which is found in about 80 to 90 percents of the cases of systemic sclerosis or scleroderma.

In his original descriptions of the clinical picture in 1862 as well as in 1874, Raynaud concluded that the excessive vasoconstrictive tone observed in this particular syndrome must be of central origin. If you observe closely the manifestations of the disease, you will find them to be astonishingly similar to those of the cold pressor test. Whether the extremities are in contact with cold objects or the body is exposed to a cold environment, the fingers will turn white or show blanching, followed by cyanosis, and finally by rubor or hyperemia. Typically the fingers are found to be cold, more or less numb, and maybe covered with perspiration. During the cyanotic phase, the fingers may become very achy and clumsy in fine movements. During the recovery phase, the cyanotic areas gradually becomes red, and sometimes brilliantly so. In about 10% of the patient population suffering with Raynaud's disease, thickening and tightening of the subcutaneous tissue may develop. When these vasomotor changes occur in conjunction with other medical conditions, it is called Raynaud's phenomenon, and when it occurs primarily and independent of other medical illnesses it is called Raynaud's disease.

The Raynaud's phenomenon is sort of like a naturally occurring cold pressor test. First, when the body is subjected to cold, the arterioles supplying the fingers and hands become constrictive, causing the area to blanch. This is more or less parallel to the vasoconstrictive phase of the cold pressor test, wherein the blood pressure begins to rise. In the subsequent phase, blood then rushes towards the extremities, due to the dilatation of blood vessels supplying the extremities, and this rush of blood circulation to the area causes the area to become bright red or hyperemic. This phase is very similar to the vasodilation phase in the cold pressor test, whereas the blood pressure now drops below the baseline. And finally, a normal vascular tone is reestablished in the area, which is equivalent to the cold pressor test, and which ultimately leads to a reestablishment of the blood pressure. If you look at the curves representing the different states of kidney deficiency in Key K-5, you will see the dotted line representing the more advanced state of kidney deficiency, namely kidney yin and kidney yang deficiency. There is an exaggerated response in the rise of blood pressure, and also a prolonged depression of blood pressure below the baseline. This exaggerated biphasic pattern is quite typical in patients with Raynaud's phenomenon, leading to blanching first, followed by hyperemia. Therefore whenever Raynaud's phenomenon is observed, one can probably safely conclude that there is a significant degree of kidney deficiency. The advanced state of kidney deficiency usually is associated with yang deficiency manifestations, as well. In other words, there are more cold symptoms as opposed to hot symptoms, and this is rather easy to remember because cold actually aggravates the situation, and cold agglutinins, cryoglobulinemia, and cryofibrinogenemia are found to be associated with Raynaud's phenomenon. And beta blocker, which is a yin substance or an anti-yang substance because it blocks the sympathetic beta receptor, is known to aggravate this condition.

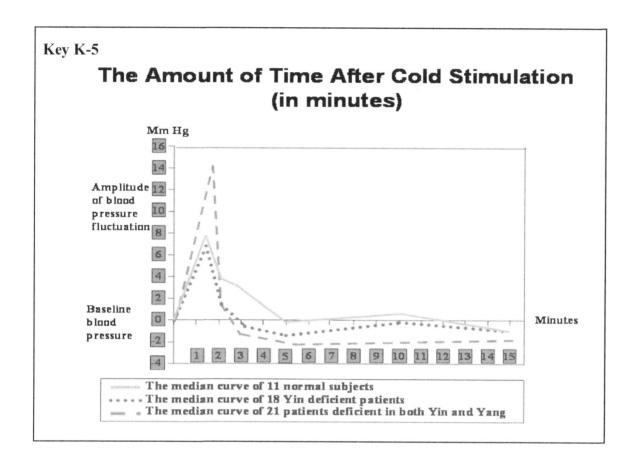

Key K-5

The Amount of Time After Cold Stimulation (in minutes)

Mm Hg

Amplitude of blood pressure fluctuation

Baseline blood pressure

Minutes

——— The median curve of 11 normal subjects
• • • • • The median curve of 18 Yin deficient patients
— — The median curve of 21 patients deficient in both Yin and Yang

So, when Raynaud's phenomenon exists, you know pretty well that you are going to get abnormal laboratory findings regarding the 17-hydroxy and 17-ketocorticosteroids during the acute phase of the disease, such as the winter. Although one can correlate well Raynaud's phenomenon with a yang deficiency state, the reverse is not necessarily true. In other words, not every yang deficient patient will have the phenomenon, and you probably have to challenge them with a cold pressor test to document that abnormal vasomotor response, other than, of course, to check their radial pulse and look at the tongue and use other diagnostic criteria.

But there is a nifty test you can perform with virtually no expense, and you don't have to wait around for the lab to report to you the result. The test is based on the phenomenon known as dermographism. Although it is not exactly equivalent to the cold pressor test, it does give very useful clinical information as to the state of the patient, whether he or she is yin or yang deficient, or more likely deficient in both. Dermo means skin and graph means picture. So if you draw on the skin and a picture results, the patient has dermographism. To do this test, you simply stroke along the skin with a blunt instrument or object such as the edge of a coin or even your fingernail somewhat vigorously but not enough to cause any actual breakage of the skin. Soon after you have done that, you will notice a little line of erythema along the course of the stroking, which if positive for dermographism, will soon turn into a bumpy line due to wheal formation, and finally there is a macular erythematous area surrounding this line. This triad of red line, wheal formation.

119

and flare is known as the triple response of Lewis, as outlined in Key K-12. The triple response of Lewis is a normal response of normal skin to this mechanical stimulus.

Key K-12

Triple Response of Lewis

1. Red Line

2. Wheal

3. Flare

The usefulness of this test comes in when the dermographic response deviates from normal, and there are two types of abnormalities. One abnormal response is that after being stroked, the area first appears to be red. This red line at the stroke site will soon be replaced by a white line, and a surrounding blanched area. A wheal also fails to form. This reaction is therefore considered different from the expected triple response of Lewis, and is known as white dermographism. This phenomenon is frequently observed in patients suffering from various kinds of dermatitis, such as the atopic dermatitis, and this technique has been applied to an area of active dermatitis. This reaction can be considered as a sub-normal response of dermographism because the skin seems to have failed to react to this outside challenge.

Swings to the other side of the spectrum, the other type of abnormal responses consist of an exaggerated response or an overreaction to this mechanical stimulation. In this instance, dermographism is an elevated edematous response occurring along the line of external application of pressure with a dull pointed object, and this elevated line may persist for a while. This type of dermographism is frequently found in patients suffering from chronic urticaria.

So how do these two types of dermographism fit into the scheme of TCM, and how are they related to what we have just discussed? Well, the sub-normal response found in atopic dermatitis is closely related to the yang deficient state. The symptoms of asthma and eczema are often associated with the syndrome of coldness, a yang deficient-yin excessive state. The formation of the white line or prolonged blanching is associated with constriction of the micro-circulation supplying that area. Urticaria, on the other hand, is considered in TCM as having too much wind and heat, a yang excess-yin deficiency state. So by simply stroking an area of the skin and observing the dermographic changes, you might be able to gain some valuable clinical insight into the condition of that patient without a lot of fancy lab work. The test is easily performed by using the handle of your percussion hammer as you would test for a Babinski sign, or even using your fingernail.

This test is especially handy when you check an area of pathology. For example, a patient is suffering from middle back pain, let's say around the level of T10. So you may want to examine the skin condition in the neighborhood of the pathology, and you may want to do a test of dermographism in this particular area. If any abnormal response is elicited, you know in what direction the pathology had shifted, whether towards the yin excess or the yang excess state, and you will be able to devise a treatment plan that would overcome this abnormal shift. Again, the subnormal as well as exaggerated response of dermographism has something to do with the altered vascular reactions, in some way similar but not identical to the cold pressor response or the Raynaud's phenomenon.

The mechanical stimulation leading to the formation of the wheal may be associated with the release of histamine into the area. In a normal person, intradermal injection of histamine also results in a wheal and flare, but in areas of atopic dermatitis, there is a wheal but little or no flare. Also, normally, intradermal injection of acetylcholine causes a wheal and a flare, but in sites of active atopic dermatitis, the flare is replaced by a few minutes of blanching. The flare will also be absent when the cutaneous nerve supplying the area has been cut. This shows the vascular response is really controlled by the nerves, which in turn, are directly related to the global functions of the yin and yang neurons in the CNS, as we had discussed earlier.

The reason we are spending time studying the vasomotor functions of the vascular system is because the behavior of the vascular system closely reflects what the CNS is doing. The measurement of blood pressure in modern medicine, the palpation of various pulses in the body in a discipline known as pulse diagnosis in traditional Chinese medicine, which has been studied extensively by generations after generations of TCM practitioners, as well as Dr. Nogier's study on the vascular autonomic signal or VAS, in auricular medicine which extends beyond ear acupuncture, are all excellent examples of diagnostic techniques involving the observation of cardiovascular changes to derive an understanding of the how the CNS functions in a particular disease state. In other words, when the CNS functions abnormally in various kidney deficiency states, it will definitely affect the behavior of the vasomotor functions.

When a normal healthy subject exercises, his coronary arteries will dilate, supplying more oxygen to the cardiac muscles, but this is not the case for somebody who has coronary artery disease, as vigorous exercise may induce constriction of the coronary vessels, leading to ischemic symptoms. If acetylcholine is applied to a normal section of artery, including that of the coronary arteries, vasodilatation will be induced. Norepinephrine, on the other hand, will cause vasoconstriction.

In a series of experiments that ultimately led to the winning of the Nobel Prize, it was found that the endothelium of the arteries will produce paradoxical vasoconstriction when stimulated with acetylcholine. And as it turns out, the endothelium is responsible for the production of a chemical substance later known as EDRF, or endothelium derived relaxing factor, which produces vasodilatation in all sorts of arteries, both in humans and in animals. And, when arteries are diseased as in the case of atherosclerosis, these vessels have a proclivity to contract or constrict, leading to ischemia. This substance was later on identified as nitric oxide, of course; it also plays a vital role in the workings of sildenafil, more commonly known as Viagra, which interferes with the enzyme phosphodiesterase, making more nitric oxide available, inducing a dilatation of the sinusoid in the penis as well as in the arterial supply, achieving its therapeutic function in the treatment of impotence.

One of the six disease entities we listed in Key K-3 is atherosclerosis which, of course, is frequently associated with angina and erectile dysfunctions reflecting the abnormal behavior of the blood vessels. From the traditional Chinese medicine point of view, these conditions are affiliated with kidney deficiency, oftentimes kidney yin deficiency, which can be helped by Chinese herbal agents as well as acupuncture therapeutics. This is why acupuncture is beneficial in the treatment of both cardiac ischemia, as well as erectile dysfunction; EDRF can be considered a yin substance because it counterbalances the actions of norepinephrine and other sympathomimetic neural hormones. The production of EDRF or nitric oxide may indeed be quite impaired in kidney deficiency states, leading to exaggerated vasomotor responses, including an exaggerated vasoconstrictive phase initially, as in the cold pressor test.

Key K-3

<u>Some Clinical Entities of
Kidney Qi Deficiency</u>

- Bronchial asthma
- Anovulatory functional uterine bleeding
- Discoid or systemic lupus erythematosus
- Chronic fatigue syndrome
- Coronary atherosclerosis
- Toxemia of pregnancy

In the practice of acupuncture, even if you were to limit your practice to the treatment of pain alone, you would find many of your patients have comorbid conditions such a hypertension, diabetes, coronary heart disease, heart failure, chronic fatigue syndrome, etc., etc., etc. And if you fail to appreciate the pathophysiological undertow in these patients, you will not be effective in helping these patients with their chronic pain, because it is these very conditions that predispose them to develop their painful conditions in the first place. So your therapeutic objective is to shift the balance of your patient back to normal as much as possible, and the therapeutic outcome will be much better.

Another important point to remember here is that myocardial infarction is often not the result of a plumbing problem. In other words, it is not the progressive clogging of the artery that led to the heart attack, because the majority of MIs occur in patients with less than 50% patency. It happened because there was a fissure in the fibrous cap causing the formation of a thrombus that occluded the artery; such events are often heralded by vasospasm. MI occurs a lot often in the morning because of the rising titer of catecholamines in the morning hours. Stress is another important factor, whether it is physical stress from overexertion during sexual activity, or stress resulting from emotional upheaval.

They all have something in common: the increased sympathetic tone is equivalent to the traditional Chinese concept of mobilizing yang, leading to vasoconstriction and spasm, causing the destruction of the plaque, thereby initiating the cascade of events that ultimately leads to coronary artery occlusion. So we can view the plaque as a necessary condition for MI, but not necessary the sufficient condition and the sufficient condition is mediated by neural impulses that originate from the brain. So it is not surprising at all that acupuncture is capable of relieving the symptoms of angina, since acupuncture works on the central nervous system, which mediates these adverse physiological events. The statin drugs are known to decrease cardiovascular events long before there is evidence of any thinning of the plaque in the arteries, and there is no reason why that this class of drugs cannot be administered with a TCM herbal formula, along with treatment with acupuncture, to intercept or even reverse the pathological process of atherosclerosis. And I venture to predict that sometime in the future, a double-blind randomized control study will prove this, and the practice of TCM will change the landscape of modern medicine permanently.

Chapter Nine – Applying TCM Principles in the Modern Clinical Setting

If all of a sudden your visual acuity for one particular color, let's say red or green, were to become heightened, you'd begin to see patterns you hadn't recognized before, and you would have increased perception for a particular type of reality.

Now that you have some working knowledge about yin and yang, let's have you put on a pair of glasses, a pair of "polarized" glasses to give you a much keener vision of yin and yang, so you will gain new insight into the practice of modern medicine. As I've said before, the whole world can be classified into the yin and yang components. That means there are yin and yang infectious agents, there are yin and yang antibiotics, there are yin and yang drugs, there are yin and yang personalities, there are yin and yang food items, there are yin and yang constitutions, yin and yang diseases, and so on and so forth.

So let us take a good look around and see what we can see. Let's take a look at some of the common lab tests, and see if we can make heads or tails about what they represent.

CBC, hemoglobin, and hematocrit: If they are decreased, we know the body is in some kind of trouble. According to traditional Chinese medicine, the body is nothing more than blood and qi. Blood is a yin substance and qi is yang, and when the blood component is compromised, the body is in the state of disharmony. Let's say the anemia is microcytic and microchromic due to a lack of dietary iron, then, of course the problem can be promptly corrected with iron supplement.

But in many clinical situations, the cause of the anemia cannot be determined, the so-called anemia associated with chronic diseases. It is as if the body is so busy fighting off the disease that it does not have enough time or energy to make more red blood cells. When this is encountered, one would know that the blood and qi in this patient are depleted. This is easily ascertainable by ordering a simple blood test. But of course, in ancient times, TCM practitioners had only their clinical acumen and diagnostic skills to rely on.

This concept of deficiency of blood and qi can also account for the finding of anemia in older patients, where a definite cause for the lower hematocrit and hemoglobin may not be found. Conversely, polycythemia is a condition associated with excessive amounts of qi and blood, or a state of congestion rather than deficiency. The statistically higher amount of hemoglobin in men versus women is due to the stimulatory effect of testosterone, which can be considered in TCM as a qi and blood tonifier.

Based on the lab result of anemia, one can safely conclude that the yin component of that patient is deficient. Although yin deficiency can coexist with yang deficiency as we have pointed out earlier, this patient is, at the minimum, yin deficient.

Because of the yin deficiency, you may observe a relative yang excess, or what I call the pseudo-yang phenomenon. The patient may have a pink flush in the face, giving rise to a false impression on others that this person is in relatively good health, mimicking an individual with copious amounts of qi and blood, indicative of good health. Upon closer examination with all the other diagnostic techniques, one will find that they are not, in fact, healthy, and we will talk more about that in the workshop on diagnostics.

What about the white cell count? Well, this is a bit trickier because not all white cells are alike. A high white count with a shift to the left consisting of a higher number of polymorphonucleocytes is generally indicative of excessive yang, and more likely than not represents a congestive state as in many acute infections, such as acute pharyngitis, pneumonia and meningitis, and so on. But if eosinophilia is found, that patient is most likely suffering from a more severe kidney deficiency state, and much more often associated with a cold syndrome. It is well established that eosinophilia is often associated with various kinds of allergic reactions, such as infestations with parasites like roundworms, hookworms and the like, and other non-infectious entities such as collagen diseases.

In my clinical experience, I have found that many patients suffering from multiple allergies, such as multiple chemical sensitivities, also experience many symptoms and show signs of severe kidney deficiency, and as the underlying kidney deficiency gets corrected, even partially, they become less allergic across the board, as if there exists somewhere in the body a "global allergy stat", which can up-regulate or down-regulate their overall sensitivities to various allergens. In general, the more kidneys deficient they are, the more allergic they will become. As we recall from the study of the kidney deficiency complex, the more advanced state of deficiency is characterized by a more unstable system of yin and yang balance, and the system tends to overreact.

Furthermore, this advanced kidney deficiency state is more likely to show signs of yang deficiency or the coldness syndrome. And this is exactly why eosinophilia is often linked to the coldness syndrome -- because it represents a more advanced state of kidney deficiency. Eosinophilia is associated with adrenal insufficiency syndrome. As we said earlier, the adrenals are part of the TCM kidney system. So, it is without question that adrenal insufficiency represents an advanced state of kidney qi deficiency, particularly kidney yang deficiency. Hence, it is not surprising at all to find eosinophilia.

Glucocorticoid is of course a product of the adrenal glands, and many eosinophilia-affiliated conditions can be treated successfully with glucocorticoid because it will tonify the kidney system. For instance, a *subset of* patients suffering from chronic bronchitis, which produces a large number of eosinophils in the sputum or the bronchial secretions, tends to respond very well to glucocorticoid treatment. Bronchial asthma, another typical case of kidney qi deficiency and oftentimes a cold condition, will also respond well to glucocorticoid. Eosinophilia is of course, commonly associated with bronchial asthma.

Another heterogeneous group of medical disorders known as the idiopathic hypereosinophilic syndrome has the common feature of prolonged eosinophilia of unknown cause, accompanied by organ systems' dysfunction, including the heart, central nervous system, kidneys, lungs, GI tract and the skin, even the bone marrow. The most severe complications involve the heart and the central nervous system. Löffler's syndrome is one of such conditions, and may lead to endocardial fibrosis, thrombosis, and restrictive endomyocardiopathy. All of these are manifestations of cold syndromes, and again not surprisingly, remission can be induced by the use of glucocorticoid, the kidney system tonifier which possesses many of the yang qualities. By the same reasoning, interleukin-2, a cytokine that induces eosinophilia, may be regarded as a cold substance, or a yin agent in this context.

To illustrate this concept further, let me quote you an actual case. This was a 10-year old boy who suffered from acute onset of headaches, which were rather severe. As you well know, headaches are relatively uncommon in children. So the worry was whether this boy was suffering from something ominous such as a brain tumor. Hence a CAT scan of the brain was done, and it showed no abnormal findings. But the peripheral blood showed a markedly elevated eosinophil count. The patient also suffered from GI symptoms consisting of frequent bouts of vomiting, as well as abdominal cramps. After extensive consultation with a specialist at one of the leading medical centers, the diagnosis of idiopathic eosinophilic gastroenteritis was made.

But what could be done for the patient? "Not much," was the answer. Since the condition was idiopathic, which means the docs don't know what the heck is going on, there was no specific treatment. A more detailed history-taking revealed that less than a week before the onset of the severe headaches, he was playing a soccer game in the western part of Golden Gate Park, which is in San Francisco closer to the Pacific Ocean, on a foggy and windy Saturday. And since the symptoms and signs, as well as the history, were consistent with a cold syndrome, an attempt was then made to treat his problem with a TCM approach. Wu Zhu Yu Tang, a well-known herbal formula to treat cold syndromes was prescribed.

There are four basic ingredients in this potion. They are wu zhu yu, an extremely hot substance in TCM, not prescribed until you are absolutely sure that the patient suffers from a cold syndrome. Otherwise, you may *cause* a problem by shifting the balance in the wrong direction; if the patient suffers from a yang or yin deficient condition, it would be too hot an herb. This herb is also accompanied by Ginseng, not the American Ginseng, but the Chinese variety, because it possesses different therapeutic activities. Included in the formula are also ten large red dates, and specifically, an abundance of raw ginger, up to 30 milligrams. One of the unique features of this formula is the much larger-than-usual quantity of raw ginger deployed in an herbal formula. After taking three packages in three days, the symptoms disappeared completely, never to return. And how much did the medicine cost? It was $1.50 per package, so 3 packages, or $4.50, and that was in the early 1980's. The CT scan was several hundred dollars, not even counting the consultations with the various specialists.

It was this particular case that prompted me to think about cold syndrome when eosinophilia is a prominent feature. Subsequently, I did a literature search, and realized there was indeed a strong association between the cold syndrome and eosinophilia. Otherwise, I would not suggest you automatically treat the patient as having a cold syndrome whenever you see eosinophilia.

Now let us turn our attention momentarily to the electrolytes. One of the most important electrolytes of the body is, of course, sodium. Sodium, being the main cation in the extracellular fluid, is largely responsible for it osmolality. Now the interesting question to ask is whether sodium is related more to the yang or the yin force of the body. To try to resolve this question; let's look at this question first from the theoretical point of view, and then from the practical point of view.

To illustrate our approach, let's use the renin angiotensin aldosterone system as our frame of reference. The more active this system, the higher the amount of sodium that is going to be reabsorbed, the higher the blood volume that will be circulating, and the higher the blood pressure will be. So applying the concepts of TCM, this is really a process belonging to the yang component, so we can say, sodium is a yang substance.

Water on the other hand, or pure water, is a yin element, as compared to fire, which is a yang element according to traditional Chinese medicine theories. Now let's try to correlate this theoretical framework with actual clinical observations.

Several important clinical entities such as congestive heart failure, cirrhosis of the liver, and nephrotic syndrome are often associated with severe edematous state, which is caused by volume expansion, leading to hyponatremia. In other words, there is more water than there is sodium. So under these circumstances, the body is much more yin than yang, because it has more water than it has sodium, and therefore hyponatremia is consistent with a yang deficiency state. Not only that, but according to the literature of modern medicine, the degree of hyponatremia often correlates very well with the severity of the underlying conditions, and can in fact serve as a prognosticating factor.

And now if you refer back to the chart of progression of diseases, in terms of yin and yang, you will notice yang deficiency often represents advanced stage of kidney qi deficiency. So, the greater the degree of hyponatremia, the greater the degree of yang deficiency, and the greater the degree of kidney qi deficiency, the worse the prognosis. Here the eastern medical concepts and western medical concepts coincide perfectly.

The clinical examples we have now just quoted represent the so-called hypervolemic state, where excessive amounts of fluid have been retained. So what about the normal volemic or euvolemic state, where there is a normal amount of extracellular fluid? Well, one of the most common examples of hyponatremia in euvolemic state is known as SIADH, or the syndrome of inappropriate antidiuretic hormone. The important function of the antidiuretic hormone is, of course to reabsorb as much free water as possible so that it is not lost in the urine. That is why it is called anti-diuretic.

Its action is inappropriate if there is already sufficient water inside the body, hence no need to retain more water. Yet, it keeps on working overtime in performing its functions, causing more water to be retained, causing more dilution of the blood, leading to hyponatremia, and inappropriately so. That is why it is called the syndrome of inappropriate ADH, which is found to be associated with neuropsychiatric diseases, pulmonary diseases, tumors, surgery, drugs, CNS diseases and, interestingly, porphyria.

Porphyria, a metabolic disease, is sometimes confused with Addison's Disease, because of its increased pigmentation, hyponatremia, muscle weakness, and abdominal pain.

Addison's Disease is of course characterized by kidney qi deficiency, especially kidney yang deficiency. So it comes as no surprise that an infusion of glucose intravenously actually helps these patients in their acute attacks of intermittent pophyria.

Anticonvulsants, on the other hand, tend to aggravate the attack because anticonvulsants are considered to be yin agonists, or anti-yang substances, which will push the body in the wrong direction. In SIADH, the natremia-stat, or the control of the blood sodium, is set low, even though the patient is euvolemic. This low natremia setting is commonly associated with various kinds of pathological processes. For example, in cachexia and malnutrition, obviously kidney qi deficiency states, the "osmo-stat" in the brain is down-regulated, causing hyponatremia. Cancer cells are also known to produce anti-diuretic hormone ectopically, and different kinds of carcinomas, especially tumors of the lung, are capable of producing the anti-diuretic hormone, which down-regulates the "natremia-stat," resulting in hyponatremia, a yang deficiency state. And it is not surprising to find this to be the case because the lung tissue, according to TCM, belongs to a very yin organ.

Other conditions such as hypoxemia, hypercarbia, or too much carbon dioxide in the blood, which can be characterized as yin conditions, are also known to be associated with SIADH or hyponatremia. Hyponatremia is of course not always associated with SIADH. Other forms of hormonal imbalances found in adrenal insufficiency and hypothyroidism can also lead to hyponatremia, without the involvement of the syndrome of inappropriate ADH. Once again, adrenal insufficiency and hypothyroidism are quite typical of yang deficiency, and believe it or not, people drinking too much beer can also lead to hyponatremia. The current modern medical explanation is that these people do not eat properly, therefore they do not obtain enough sodium, and that is why they can be hyponatremic. The condition is known as beer potomania because they are crazy about drinking beer. From the analysis of traditional Chinese medicine, however, beer is about the most yin kind of alcoholic drink. Therefore, if you subscribe to the notion of TCM, you should advise the patient not to drink too much beer if they are found to be yang deficient or having symptomatology relating to a cold syndrome.

Now what if the pendulum swings the other way, that the patient instead of having hyponatremia has hypernatremia? A patient may, of course, suffer from hypernatremia if fluid is withheld or inaccessible, or has been having a high intake of salt on a temporary basis. These problems can be corrected quickly and should not be the focus of our current attention. What we are talking about is essential hypernatremia. In other words, the natremia-stat is now set high instead of low. On a chronic basis, if hyponatremia is considered to be a yin condition, should we then say, hypernatremia is associated with a yang condition? According to the authoritative medical text by Harrison, patients suffering from essential? diabetes insipidus, caused by a lack of action by the antidiuretic hormone vasopressin, leading to an excessive loss of free water via the urine, resulting in the blood being more concentrated in solutes including sodium, hence, hypernatremia will not only have the symptoms of polyuria and thirst, but also for some unknown reason, "These patients would prefer the drinking of ice-cold water, not simply just drinking fluid to quench their thirst."

Well, according to the scheme of TCM, this is easily explainable because those patients who are having too much yang energy in the body, also have the tendency to have a hot syndrome. Therefore, they prefer to drink cold water; we have already talked about that in the kidney yin deficiency state, listed in the table in Key K-10. A preference for cold drinks is prototypical of kidney yin deficiency, which is equivalent to a relatively typically yang excess state.

Key K-10

Summary of Symptoms, Signs and Kidney Deficiency Types of 17 Cases of Scleroderma

Kidney Deficiency		Kidney Yang Deficiency		Kidney Yin Deficiency	
Symptoms:	**# of Cases**	**Symptoms:**	**# of Cases**	**Symptoms:**	**# of Cases**
Backache back tiredness	10	Aversion to cold & cold extremities	13	Dizziness	4
Weak extremities	4	Cold feeling on back	3	Visual disturbance	4
Heel pain	3	Spontaneous sweating	3	Small voiding of dark urine	2
Tinnitus	5	Preference for hot drinks	6	Constipation	3
Hearing loss	3	Sexual impotence	3	Insomnia	3
Premature greying of hair	1	Decreased libido	1	Night sweat	5
Loose teeth	4	Numbness in extremities	8	Nocturnal emission	1
Menstrual Irregularities	8	Large voidings of clear urine	3	Preference for cold drinks	1
		Nocturia	3		
Signs		Pale or dusty Complexion	8	**Signs**	
Weak chueh pulse (proximal radial pulse)	16			Faint pulse	5
		Signs		Soft or slippery pulse	4
		Pulse small & lax	6	Bow pulse	2
		Bulky & delicate looking tongue	12	Tip + side of tongue red	2
		Teeth marks	14	Central fissures	3
				Central patches without coating	1

Hypernatremia is also associated with increased risk of subarachnoid and intracranial hemorrhage, and these are indeed signs of excessive yang, according to TCM. Other symptoms such as neuromuscular irritability, seizures, rather typical of the yang excess symptomatology are also found in hypernatremia.

Another important electrolyte is, of course, potassium. Potassium always seems to play on the other side of sodium. Sodium is primarily an extracellular fluid component, whereas potassium is found mainly in the intracellular compartment. The action of the hormone aldosterone is to exchange the two ions by absorbing the sodium and excreting the potassium.

So the interesting question arises: Whether potassium functions in a way somewhat opposite to sodium, which is a yang substance.

Again, according to current medical literature, epidemiological studies have linked a low potassium diet with increased incidences of essential hypertension, which will respond to treatment by potassium supplementation in the diet. But the pathophysiological mechanism of how this whole thing works is currently unclear. But here is something for us to think about: We know a high sodium diet can also cause the blood pressure to rise, because sodium is a yang substance. If we think of potassium as a yin substance, then a lack of yin can also cause the blood pressure to rise, just like an excess of yang. Some of our patients may be on diuretics, and we ask them to replenish potassium by drinking orange juice or eating bananas because they are rich in potassium. But it so happens that according to TCM, these dietary substances are also cold substances or substances that are predominately yin in nature. According to this scheme, the intake of potassium probably will push the body towards the yin direction, so we can see that any drug that shifts the balance towards retention of potassium probably will have the same effect.

Take the example of Triamterene or Spironolactone, the so-called potassium-sparing diuretics. Their main action is to work against aldosterone, the hormone that is a yang-agonist, as we have previously discussed. So these are yin substances that will result in retention of potassium, making the body more yin. So there is little wonder that eosinophilia, a hallmark of cold syndrome in most instances, is one of the side-effects of these drugs, due to their yin nature.

Now, having looked at these fascinating applications of TCM concepts in western medicine, we need to insert a cautionary note here. We cannot rely on just the blood level of a certain element to draw a conclusion as to whether the patient is suffering from a yang excess or yin excess condition; we must also incorporate other diagnostic techniques to accomplish the clinical assessment of that patient. For example, the total of the body's potassium may not be expressed by the blood level alone, due to the fact that potassium is found mainly in the intracellular compartment. So when a patient with diabetic ketoacidosis is treated with insulin, the blood level of potassium will be shifted downward quickly, because it is transferred from the extracellular fluid compartment into the intracellular compartment, and one should not rely on a single parameter to reach a clinical diagnosis.

Take the example of thyroid stimulating hormone or TSH. Due to the symptomatology of Grave's Disease or hyperthyroidism, we know the thyroid hormone is a yang substance. So TSH must necessarily be yang also, because it is the commander of the thyroid. It is the thyroid agonist or yang agonist, so to speak. But if you simply look at the blood level of TSH and say to yourself, "If TSH is a yang substance, a high level of TSH must mean that the patient is suffering from a yang excess condition," it goes without saying that if you do that, you will be absolutely wrong. So when you use the yin and yang concept, or later on, the five elements concept to evaluate the effect of therapy or assess the condition of the patient, you must not be fooled by the tunnel vision of focusing only on one aspect of the problem. Nonetheless, I think this exercise of using the TCM concept to analyze our day-to-day clinical experience is an extremely valuable one, and will definitely help us to put everything that we do into proper perspective, enabling us to follow certain lines of thought in ways that were never possible before. Many clinical observations are like stars in the sky, which appear to be totally chaotic to the untrained eye, while in fact, their distribution follows a strict cosmic order, governed by simple yet elegant laws of physics.

And the yin and yang concept in Chinese medicine is but one of many useful concepts that will permit a more orderly way of thinking in modern medicine.

Now let us turn our attention to the more commonly ordered blood tests. Serum creatinine and the level of BUN are two common tests for renal functions, although the 24 hour creatinine clearance test is really a better test, but it is clumsier to perform and is much less convenient for the patient.

When these indicators are up, of course we know something wrong is brewing in the kidneys. When this happens, there is no question that there is a kidney deficiency state, according to TCM, because now the kidney system is not only physiologically involved, but anatomically involved, and the kidney deficiency state has to have been in existence for some time. But the reverse is not necessarily true. In other words, when there are symptoms and signs of kidney qi deficiency, whether it is kidney yang or kidney yin qi deficiency, the kidney organ may not have been involved, although the kidney *system* is implicated. Under these circumstances, the kidney function tests may be entirely normal. So the kidney function tests are really of positive predictive value. In other words, when it is positive, it means kidney deficiency, when it is negative, it doesn't mean anything as far as the system of kidney qi is concerned.

What about hyperbilirubinemia, which according to modern medical science, is divided into the conjugated and the unconjugated fractions, whose respective elevations may help distinguish the obstructive and the non-obstructive types of jaundice? Traditional Chinese medicine, as practiced thousands of years ago, did not have the luxury of modern lab work, so it looks at jaundice with a jaundiced eye. What I mean is that it will use the color to distinguish different types of jaundice. There is yin jaundice, and there is yang jaundice. Yin jaundice is associated with a dull color. It is lackluster and appears duskier, and the balance of the symptom-complex is yin dominant. Whereas, yang jaundice is manifested by a bright yellow or livelier yellow, which is accompanied by a symptom-complex of yang excess. Both conditions share a common denominator. That is, spleen or pancreatic deficiency is a hallmark. The concept of pancreatic deficiency will be discussed later.

To put it simply, the function of the spleen or pancreas is a symbol for the digestive system. As we shall see later, the word spleen in traditional Chinese medicine is a misnomer as it actually represents the pancreas. The pancreatic system, or spleen, dislikes wetness or moisture. And both the yin jaundice and the yang jaundice states are characterized by too much wetness in the pancreatic system. So yang jaundice is wet and hot, and yin jaundice is cold and wet. Yang jaundice tends towards acute, and yin jaundice towards chronic. Jaundice due to acute hepatitis is likely to be yang jaundice, and jaundice secondary to, let's say, liver cirrhosis, is likely to be yin jaundice. Jaundice as a result of hemolytic anemia may be yin or yang jaundice, although quite a different number of hemolytic anemias are related to coldness or a yang-deficient state, and in these instances, the clinical manifestation is that of yin jaundice. Although there is really no good treatment in western medicine for adults suffering from jaundice, there are specific herbal therapies in Chinese medicine and likewise in acupuncture or moxibustion, to accelerate its clearance.

Since wetness is the culprit in all jaundice conditions, one excellent way of getting rid of jaundice is through the urinary system. Various herbal agents are known to promote diuresis. Since the herbal agents used for diuresis in traditional Chinese medicine are not the same diuretic agents used in modern medicine, it is unknown at this time whether diuretic agents such as Furosemide? or Hydrochlorothiazide may actually accelerate the clearance of jaundice in patients, suffering from, say, acute hepatitis. The concept can quite easily be tested in hospitalized patients suffering from acute hepatitis. Since the treatment for acute hepatitis is mainly supportive, and both the doctors and patients are basically playing a waiting game until the symptoms spontaneously go away, one can perhaps design a clinical investigation consisting of three groups of patients, one group receiving placebo; the second group receiving a modern diuretic, and then the third group receiving the conventional Chinese herbal formula. The clinical course of these patients can be followed closely, with their symptoms well documented and the objective physical findings such as jaundice being measured over the course of time, so that we will know for sure whether the traditional Chinese formula is effective, whether the modern diuretic is also effective and if so, if it is effective to the same degree, and to establish once and for all whether diuresis alone can shorten the duration of an illness such as hepatitis A, and what might be the exact physiological mechanism through which the clearance of bilirubin can be accelerated.

In the famous medical book called Important Strategies of the Golden Chest (Jin Kui Yao Lue) authored by Zhang Zhong Jing in Eastern Han Dynasty approximately 1800 years ago, jaundice was classified into five types, namely, the yellow jaundice, grain or dietary jaundice, alcoholic jaundice, sex-related jaundice and dark jaundice, but for our present discussion, the yang jaundice and yin jaundice are quite sufficient for the purpose of illustrating the two most basic therapeutic approaches.

Next, what is the significance of the liver enzymes such as SGOT and SGPT, now known as AST and ALT? The elevation of these enzymes usually signifies hepatocellular injury, and since the liver is considered a highly reactive organ, the elevation of these indicators usually relates to a yang excessive state, or a pseudo-yang excess state.

Assuming you have a good foundation in TCM, one of the major advantages of doing TCM as a physician trained in modern medicine is that through our western training, we have acquired the ability to recognize many disease entities which have been well described in modern medical literature. The symptoms, the signs, the pathophysiology, the clinical course, the prognosis and so on, have been worked out in detail, even though in many instances, we are not able to do anything for the patient, in terms of treatment. But having acquired these theoretical tools of traditional Chinese medicine, we can use these tools to analyze what we have learned about the diseases in terms of western modern science, and obtain a clear orientation as to which therapeutic direction one must take. At the same time, it makes much more sense out of what we are doing in modern medical practice, even though none of the TCM techniques such as acupuncture or herbal therapy have been applied. So let us focus our attention on a couple of dermatological conditions, in order to illustrate what I have just said. I am using skin diseases as the first example, because both the skin and the brain are derived from the ectoderm embryologically, and many central nervous system dysfunctions are associated with manifestations of changes in the skin, which are of course easily observable with the naked eye.

Let's first turn our attention to the recurrent staphylococcal infections of the skin. Many of these patients have bacteria in their nasopharynx, or in other words, they are chronic carriers of staphylococci in the nasopharynx. If this carrier state is not eliminated, there is the obvious reason why the skin can be re-infected -- because the organism can be seeded on the skin from the nasopharynx. So for these conditions, a combination of dicloxacillin and rifampin is used. The addition of rifampin is due to the fact that refampin is concentrated many times in the nasal secretion. So when it is used in combination with the other antibiotics, such dicloxacillin, it has a greater potential of eliminating the organisms.

So far, everything is fine and dandy because everything is quite explainable within the context of western medicine. And now comes a very intriguing and interesting study performed by investigators in Israel. This study included a total of 41 patients with recurrent infections in the skin, such as recurrent folliculosis, and out of these 41 patients, 18 of them had positive staphylococcus culture in the nasopharynx. For the remaining 23 patients, one gram of vitamin C per day was administered for six weeks.

Prior to the treatment, these patients were tested for abnormal neutrophil functions, such as phagocytosis, superoxide generation, or chemotaxis. It was found that 12 out of these 23 patients had abnormal neutrophil functions, and the other 11 had normal functions of their neutrophils.

So what happened after six weeks of vitamin C therapy? Among the 12 subjects with abnormal neutrophil functions, 10 of them regained their neutrophil functions after the six weeks of vitamin C therapy, and they remained normal from one to three years in terms of their neutrophil functions, as well as absence of staphylococcus infections. The remaining two patients were also helped by vitamin C but in their cases, they had to continue using vitamin C, and if they stopped using it, they would experience a relapse of staph infections. The other 11 patients who had no abnormal functions with their neutrophils to begin with were not helped by vitamin C.

Another observation made by the investigators was that patients who benefited from the vitamin C therapy actually had a lower serum level of vitamin C prior to the therapy itself, and after six weeks or so of treatment, even though no further vitamin C was administered, the vitamin C blood level returned to normal baseline.

These very intriguing experimental results are explained by the authors in the following manner: As the neutrophils performed their functions, they auto-oxidized their cell membranes, which made them less effective in performing phagocytosis and chemotaxis, making them less effective against the infectious agents. So the more tired they got, the harder they worked because their cell membranes got oxidized. Vitamin C on the other hand is a free-radical scavenger, so it has the tendency to neutralize the effect of the oxidation of the cell membrane. So it really has a rejuvenating effect on the cell membrane, enabling the neutrophils to fulfill their defensive functions once more. That is why the 11 patients with normal functions of the neutrophils did not receive any therapeutic benefits from taking vitamin C.

Now we can look at the same set of experimental data from the viewpoint of TCM. According to traditional Chinese medicine, vitamin C should be considered a yin or cold substance; maybe that is why a lot of people think taking vitamin C is a cool thing to do. And staph infections including the carrier state are a hot condition. So what do the TCM principles tell us to do to treat hot conditions? Cool it. So using a cold substance such as vitamin C to counteract the problems of too much yang or too much heat in the system is quite logical.

The depleted level of vitamin C in the serum of the 12 patients who had recurrent infections with staphylococci was naturally indicative of a yang excess state, and that is why their neutrophils did not function normally. So when the cool substance of vitamin C was administered to this group of patients, it reduced the excess yang, cooling down the system, which basically prevented the recurrence of the infection. Likewise, in the practice of TCM, acupuncture or herbal treatments can be administered to cool down the system as well, and can accomplish the same therapeutic goal without antibiotics, say. The advantage of this approach is that you don't have to give the treatment all the time. Once you get the problem corrected by adjusting the system towards normalcy, you can stop all the treatments, yet the body will continue to function normally. In this case six weeks of 1 gram of vitamin C orally per day will do the trick. And the patient's physiological state, as far as the yin and yang system goes, is equivalent to the yang excess-yin deficiency state.

If you go back and revisit the diagram in Key K-9, the second column shows excess in yang and deficiency in yin in the acute phase. This column is probably representative of those 10 patients who responded nicely to the six-week course of vitamin C therapy, whereas the two other patients who required continual administration of vitamin C were more likely to be related to the group of syndromes in the third column, with a deficiency in both yin and yang, but predominantly yin deficient. So in them, the problem did not self-correct, and they needed an additional maintenance dosage of vitamin C to keep the system in balance, whereas the group of patients who did not have abnormal neutrophil functions and who did not respond positively to the vitamin C supplementation could have been a group of patients suffering from a deficiency state of both yin and yang. So we can see here that further pushing of the system into the yin direction using a cool substance such as vitamin C did not help them, or maybe they had other contributing factors not included in the present study.

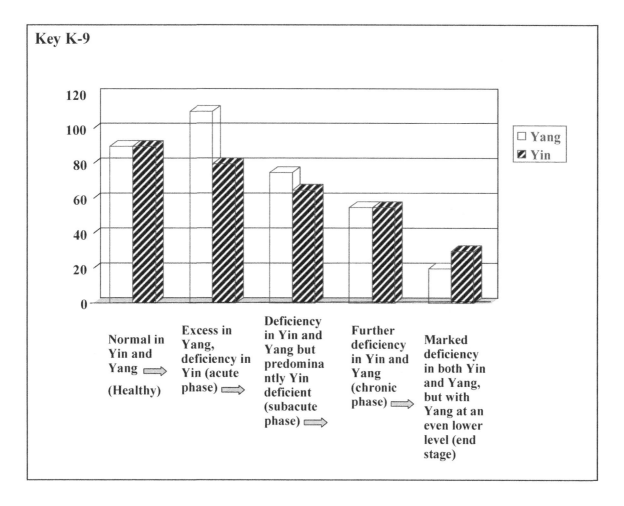

It is probably appropriate to say a few words about vitamin C at this juncture regarding its cooling properties in relation to its health benefits. Vitamin C was previously thought of as just one of the many vitamins whose function was to maintain normal physiological processes in the body. That a lack of dietary intake of vitamin C will lead to scurvy is now a well-known medical fact. But it has assumed the role of a medicine over and beyond that of an essential nutrient after Linus Pauling touted it to be a very effective agent in the treatment of the common cold, as well as for the prevention of a number of degenerative diseases, including cancer. For a while there was raging controversy in medical circles as to the validity of Linus Pauling's claim, and for a long time, mainstream medicine had poo-pooed the idea. But for the last couple of decades or so, vitamin C has come back in a big way, and conventional medicine acknowledges the benefits of vitamin C, especially its role as an antioxidant. Besides, vitamin C megadosing up to, say, 1 or 2 grams per day has been practiced by many health conscious individuals for decades, so vitamin C is a big sale item for the health food stores.

Yet in a study completed in April, 2000, a National Academy of Sciences panel proclaimed that there is no convincing scientific evidence that taking large amounts of vitamin C, vitamin E, or other nutrients can reduce the chances of getting cancer, heart disease, diabetes, Alzheimer's disease, and other illnesses. Their position was that there is insufficient evidence to recommend that the U. S. population take these nutrients, other than to prevent nutritional deficiencies. And they went on to say that extremely high doses of such supplements might lead to health problems. They recommended a mere 75 milligrams per day to be the correct level of intake for vitamin C.

How shall we reconcile the difference in opinion from all these experts?

The concept of traditional Chinese medicine can actually answer these questions in a very elegant and simple manner. In a democratic society, all men are created equal. It is, of course, a politically correct statement. But in a biological system, this belief is far from being correct. The fact that different individuals having different genetic make-ups have different tendencies towards the development of specific illnesses is well recognized in the teachings of TCM. Therefore, considering that all men are unequal, all women are unequal, and women are not equal to men (physiologically speaking that is) is standard operating procedure in TCM. The old adage, "One man's meat is another man's poison" really epitomizes this particular concept. It can be further paraphrased to say, "One man's medicine is another man's poison, and vice versa".

If you select a population at random, half of that population is likely to have the yang constitution, and the other half the yin constitution. The yang constitution group or the yang excess group is more likely to develop symptoms relating to yang excess, and the yin excess group will be more predisposed to develop symptoms of yin excess. Linus Pauling was, of course a yang individual himself; by using vitamin C in megadoses, he was able to shift his physiological parameters towards the yin direction, creating a more harmonious balance within his own body, and as a result he was less likely to get sick, including catching common colds.

But not everybody is Linus Pauling, not everybody has a hot constitution. So if you cool off the body too much by taking a megadose of vitamin C, it can produce yin symptoms, or side effects such as diarrhea. So if you were to randomly administer a cooling agent to the entire population, you will shift their physiology either towards or away from a balanced state, in effect making some of them better and the others worse.

In the U. S. population, because of the dietary intake and lifestyles, there are probably more yang individuals than there are yin individuals. Coffee and bacon in the morning, McDonald's hamburgers for lunch, and roast beef or steaks for dinner push the physiological parameters of the entire population towards the yang direction. So if you randomly select a hundred individuals, you may find 55 of them are relatively yang excessive, and the other 45 yang deficient or yin excessive.

So what happens if you give megadoses of vitamin C to all of them? Well, 55 of them will get better because they have excessive yang and the vitamin C will shift them back to normal, whereas the other 45 will tend to get worse because now their physiological parameters are shifted in an off-balance direction. To sum it up, 55 got better and 45 got worse, so you have gained a difference of ten. As a result, there is a statistical significance that this population of 100 subjects got benefit from taking the vitamin C, but the benefit is fairly small.

So, what really should happen from the therapeutic viewpoint is that the 55 hot individuals should receive a cooling agent such as vitamin C or some other equivalent, or an even better product from the Chinese herbal armamentarium, and the 45 cold individuals should receive warming agents which are amply available, again, in the pharmacopoeia of TCM. This way, you have a situation where you can get a 100% result. You warm up the cold individuals, and you cool down the hot individuals, and everybody feels better. This is, of course, the essential principle of TCM, which includes acupuncture, of course. The result of the treatment of recurrent staphylococcal infections of the skin with vitamin C has been itemized in the table in Key K-13. You may want to take a look at it now to consolidate your understanding of the therapeutic actions of vitamin C in terms of yin and yang.

Key K-13

Therapeutic Response to Vitamin C of 41 Patients with Recurrent Staph Infections of Skin

Staphylococci in nasopharynx by culture   18   not treated with Vitamin C

No Staphyloccci in nasopharyx by culture   23   treated with Vitamin C as follows:

Response to Vitamin C Group   6 weeks of

12 *Abnormal neutrophil functions*:   1 gm Vitamin C q.d

    Phagocytosis
    Superoxide generation   ⟶
    Chemotaxis

10   regain normal neutrophil functions and remain normal 1 to 3 years without recurrence of staph infections (probably Yang excess)

2   regain normal neutrophil functions temporarily, need maintenance dose (probably Yin deficient)

Low Vitamin C level   Normal Vitamin C level

No Response to Vitamin C Group   6 weeks of

     ⟶

11   Normal neutrophil functions   1 gm of Vitamin C q.d

No therapeutic effect (probably more deficient in Yin and Yang)

Another dermatological entity worth mentioning at this point to further illustrate the yin and yang concept is rosacea, or acne rosacea. But acne rosacea is not the same as acne vulgaris, because the pathological process is different. In acne, you will find polynuclear leukocytes in the lesion, whereas in rosacea, lymphocytes infiltration and granuloma in the biopsied lesions of rosacea. Rosacea is a rather common disorder affecting the central part of the face. It occurs in both men and women, though more often in women usually about age 40, and its incidence in the adult population is about 8%. There may be a facial flush or there may be rosy bumps, or a mixture of the two. The flush is caused by erythema or telangiectasia whereas the bumps can be papules or pustules. This disease is rather rare in dark skin individuals, and is rather common in fair-skinned people. So the condition has been thought to be related to sun damage. The facial flush is more common in women and the bumpy type is more common in men, although there may be a lot of overlap. The facial flush may be at first functional, in other words, there may really be no erythema. And the flushing is just like blushing -- it is temporary. And before the ultimate development of rosacea, these individuals may have the tendency for pronounced flushing in the face, and the flush may be precipitated by heat, emotion, alcohol, hot drinks or spicy foods.

Looking at this list of aggravating factors such as heat, emotion, alcohol, hot drinks, and spicy foods, what do you think this condition is due to? Is it a yang excess, or is it a yin excess condition? What about facial flushing, which is really yang energy rising to the head and face? What about radiation from the sun, which may have caused the skin damage? I do not think it is difficult at all for you to arrive at the conclusion that this is probably a condition caused by yang excess, which can be result in either yang excess or yang excess due to yin deficiency.

Consequently, this disease process's involving of the eyes is not totally unexpected. In one study conducted at the University of Vermont, 39 patients with rosacea seen at the dermatology clinic were marched down to the ophthalmology department to have their eyes checked, and it was found that not only did 85% of these patients have eye symptoms, but more surprisingly, 100% of the patients had signs of ocular involvement. All of them showed a markedly reduced tear break-up time.

Normally, oil is secreted by the Meibomian gland to help spread the tear over the eye, and for some reason this oil secretion process in rosacea patients was abnormal, and this film broke up early, as could be verified by a slit lamp examination with the use of fluorescene, and not infrequently blephoritis, iritis, chalazion and keratitis are associated with rosacea.

So rosacea is really not just a dermatological disease, but an ophthalmological disease as well. And all of these patients felt a grittiness or discomfort in their eyes, even though they may not have always been aware of it. But generally after successful treatment, they recognized in retrospect that their eyes were in fact not feeling right.

The modern medical treatment consists of three weeks of tetracyclines -- either Tetracycline, Minocycline or Doxycycline, all of them, the favorite cooling agents used in modern medicine for this hot disease. A more severe entity known as the rosacea fulminans can develop in women, usually, after a period of excessive stress. Manifested with pyoderma and explosive facial eruptions which usually heal without scarring, unlike acne, and can be successfully treated with Prednisone and Tetracycline. Due to their major stress, these patients probably have an abrupt deficiency of both kidney yin and kidney yang.

Index

References

1. Acupuncture Teaching Section of Shanghai Chinese Medical College. *Lecture Notes on Acupuncture*, Medical Forest Publisher, Hong Kong, 1972, pp.163-164.

2. Lee, T.N. The thalamic neuron theory and classical acupuncture. *Am. J. Acupuncture* : 273-282, 1978.

3. Lee, T.N. Thalamic neuron theory. A hypothesis concerning pain and acupuncture. *Medical Hypotheses* 3:113-121, 1977.

4. Lee, T.N. Thalamic neuron theory, the law of the five elements and the rhythmic method of classical acupuncture. Am. J. Acupuncture 9:217-226, 1981.

5. Kiang Chun Hua, et al.: "Combined Chinese and Modern Medical Therapy in the Treatment of "Kidney Deficiency Syndrome". Hong Kong, *Wan Yeh Publishing Company*, 1973.

6. Berges PV. Myofascial Pain Syndromes. *Postgrad Med.* 53, 161-168, 1973

7. Fairman D, Llavallol. MA. Talamic Tractotomy for the Alleviation of Intractable Pain in Cancer. *Cancer* 31, 700-707, 1973

8. Loeser JD. Neurosurgical Relief of Chronic Pain. *Postgrad Med.* 53, 115-119, 1973

9. Hassler R. "Afferent systems", *Pain.* Williams and Wikins, Baltimore, Maryland.

10. Editorial Board of "Neo-Medicine," Chung Shan Medical College: The Fundamental Theories of Chinese Medicine. Hong Kong, Health and Medicine Publishing Company, 1973

11. P. M. Toyama, M. Nishizawa, The physiological basis of acupuncture therapy, Journal of National Medical Association. 1972 September; 64(5): 397–402. *http://www.ncbi.nlm.nih.gov/pmc/articles/PMC2608746/*

12. Qian-Qian Li, Guang-Xia Shi, Qian Xu, Jing Wang, Cun-Zhi Liu, Lin-Peng Wang, Acupuncture Effect and Central Autonomic Regulation, Journal of Evidence Based Complement Alternate Medicine; 2013: 267959 *http://www.ncbi.nlm.nih.gov/pmc/articles/PMC3677642/*

13. Cheng Lu, Cheng Xiao, Gao Chen, Miao Jiang, Qinglin Zha, Xiaoping Yan, Weiping Kong, Aiping Lu, Cold and heat pattern of rheumatoid arthritis in traditional Chinese medicine: distinct molecular signatures indentified by microarray expression profiles in CD4-positive T cell, Rheumatology Int. 2012 January; 32(1): 61–68. *http://www.ncbi.nlm.nih.gov/pmc/articles/PMC3253282/*

14. Jingcheng Dong, The Relationship between Traditional Chinese Medicine and Modern Medicine, Journal of Evidence Based Complement Alternate Medicine , 2013. *http://www.ncbi.nlm.nih.gov/pmc/articles/PMC3745867/*

15. Lee, T.N. The Concept of "Kidney Deficiency". Modern Interpretation of a Traditional Chinese Medical Principle. *Am. J. Acupuncture*, Vol. 6, No. 2 April-June, 1978

16. Xingjiang Xiong, Xiaochen Yang, Wei Liu, Fuyong Chu, Pengqian Wang, and Jie Wang, Trends in the Treatment of Hypertension from the Perspective of Traditional Chinese Medicine, Journal of Evidence Based Complement Alternate Medicine, v.2013; 2013. *http://www.ncbi.nlm.nih.gov/pmc/articles/PMC3710609/*

17. Jia-ying Wang, Lu Xiao, Jing Chen, Jing-bo Zhai, Wei Mu, Jing-yuan Mao, Hongcai Shang, Potential effectiveness of traditional Chinese medicine for cardiac syndrome X (CSX): a systematic review and meta-analysis, Journal of Evidence Based Complement Alternate Medicine, 2013 *http://www.ncbi.nlm.nih.gov/pmc/articles/PMC3662595/*

18. Lixing Lao, Yi Huang, Chiguang Feng, Brian M Berman, Ming T. Tan, Evaluating Traditional Chinese Medicine Using Modern Clinical Trial Design and Statistical Methodology: Application to a Randomized Controlled Acupuncture Trial, Stat Med. 2012 March 30; 31(7): 619–627. http://www.ncbi.nlm.nih.gov/pmc/articles/PMC3116954/

19. Qinghui Que, Xiaode Ye, Quangui Su, Yan Weng, Jianfeng Chu, Lijuan Mei, Wenwen Huang, Renhui Lu, Guohua Zheng, Effectiveness of acupuncture intervention for neck pain caused by cervical spondylosis: study protocol for a randomized controlled trial, Trials. 2013; 14: 186. Published online 2013 June 22 http://www.ncbi.nlm.nih.gov/pmc/articles/PMC3700747/

20. Eric Manheimer, M.S., Susan Wieland, M.P.H., Ph.D., Elizabeth Kimbrough, M.P.H., Ph.D., Ker Cheng, Ph.D.(Cand.), and Brian M. Berman, M.D., Evidence from the Cochrane Collaboration for Traditional Chinese Medicine Therapies, Journal of Evidence Based Complement Alternate Medicine, 2009 September; 15(9): 1001–1014. http://www.ncbi.nlm.nih.gov/pmc/articles/PMC2856612/

Made in the USA
Monee, IL
09 May 2022

96098910R00083